COMPLETE GUIDEBOOK FOR YCB LEVEL 2 YOGA TTC

Yoga Wellness Instructor

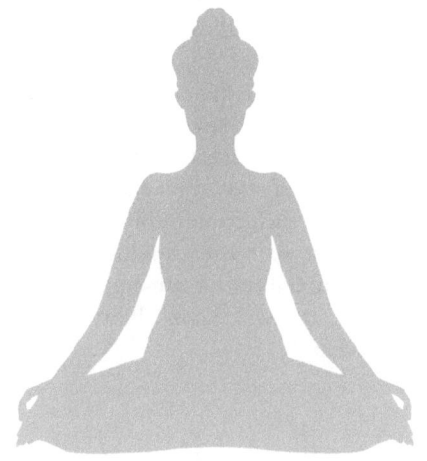

Ayushman Yog

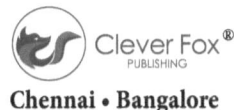

Chennai • Bangalore

CLEVER FOX PUBLISHING
Chennai, India

Published by CLEVER FOX PUBLISHING 2024
Copyright © Ayushman Yog 2024

All Rights Reserved.
ISBN: 978-93-56487-29-1

This book has been published with all reasonable efforts taken to make the material error-free after the consent of the author. No part of this book shall be used, reproduced in any manner whatsoever without written permission from the author, except in the case of brief quotations embodied in critical articles and reviews.

The Author of this book is solely responsible and liable for its content including but not limited to the views, representations, descriptions, statements, information, opinions and references ["Content"]. The Content of this book shall not constitute or be construed or deemed to reflect the opinion or expression of the Publisher or Editor. Neither the Publisher nor Editor endorse or approve the Content of this book or guarantee the reliability, accuracy or completeness of the Content published herein and do not make any representations or warranties of any kind, express or implied, including but not limited to the implied warranties of merchantability, fitness for a particular purpose. The Publisher and Editor shall not be liable whatsoever for any errors, omissions, whether such errors or omissions result from negligence, accident, or any other cause or claims for loss or damages of any kind, including without limitation, indirect or consequential loss or damage arising out of use, inability to use, or about the reliability, accuracy or sufficiency of the information contained in this book.

Atha Yoganushasanam!
"Now the journey begins"

DISCLAIMER

This textbook is a compilation of information from various sources. Ayushman Yog doesn't claim ownership of any information/source of information presented in this book. Ayushman Yog only has copyright rights to compiling the notes arranged in this book.

CONTENTS

About The Author .... *viii*
About Ayushman Yog .... *x*
Introduction .... *xi*
About The Ycb Level – 2, 400 Hrs. Yoga Ttc Exam .... *xiii*

1. Introduction To Yoga And Yogic Practices 1

1.1 Yoga: Etymology, Definition, Aim, Objectives 1
1.2 Yoga: Its origin, history, and development 11
1.3 Brief Introduction to Samkhya and Yoga Darshana 18
1.4 Life sketches and teachings of Yoga masters 26
1.5 Principles of Yoga 44
1.6 Principles and Practices of Jnana Yoga 48
1.7 Principles and Practices of Bhakti Yoga 51
1.8 Principles and Practices of Karma Yoga 52
1.9 Concept and principles of Sukshma Vyayama,
 Sthula Vyayama, Surya Namaskara, ... 53
1.10 Concept and principles of Shatkarma: 58
1.11 Concept and principles of Yogasana: 76
1.12 Concept and principles of Pranayama: 80
1.13 Introduction to Tri Bandha 91

1.14 Dhyana and its significance in health
and well-being..98
1.15 Introduction to Yogic relaxation techniques............101

2. Introduction To Yoga Text 107
2.1 Introduction to Prasthantrayi, Purushartha
Chatushtaya, and goal of human life 107
2.2 Yoga in Kathopnishad, Prashnopanishad, and
Tattiryopanishad 110
2.3 Study Of Bhagwad Gita 122
2.4 Study of Patanjali Yoga Sutra 137
2.5 Important Concept in Patanjali Yoga Sutra................146
2.6 Hatha Yoga: Parampara and Basic Yoga Texts 160
2.7 Hatha Yoga, Ref: Hatha Yoga Pradipika (HYP) 165
2.8 Hatha Yoga, Ref: Gheranda Samhita (GS)................201
2.9 Concept Of Nadi 219

3. Introduction To Yoga Text 222
3.1 General introduction to the human body 222
3.2 Introduction to sensory organs 248
3.3 Homeostasis 256
3.4 Yogic concept of health and wellness 258
3.5 Concept of Tridoshas, Sapta Dhatu, Agni,
Vayu, and Mala; 260
3.6 Dinacharya and Ritucharya 269
3.7 Importance of Ahara, Nidra, and Brahmacharya
in well-being- 273
3.8 Knowledge of common diseases; 276

4. Practical 293
   4.1 Prayer: 293
   4.2 Yogic Shat Karma: 297
   4.3 Yogic Sukshma & Sthula Vyayama 298
   4.4 Yogic Surya Namaskara 303
   4.5 Yogasana 303
   4.6 Preparatory Breathing Practices & Pranayama- 331
   4.7 Concept and Demonstration of Bandha & Mudra ... 332
   4.8 Practices Leading to Dhyan Sadhana 332
   4.9 Concept of Soham/ Hamsa 335
   4.10 Methods of Teaching & Evaluation 338

Multiple Choice Questions 346
Answers 413
Bibliography & References 417

ABOUT THE AUTHOR

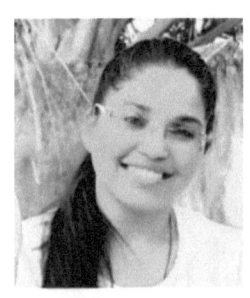

*N*idhi is the Head of the Teaching Department and a founding member of Ayushman Yog. She has been a yoga practitioner since a young age and always had a thing for learning. As her practice progressed, her curiosity for learning more about Yogic science grew stronger, she eventually did her **Level -1 Yoga Teachers Training Course** from Nityam Yoga Institute. The amazing teachers of Nityam encouraged her to see Yoga in its true essence, beyond the asanas. This led her to study traditional scriptures such as Patanjali Yoga Sutra, Hatha Yoga Pradipika, and Gheranda Samhita.

Yogic science is so vast that the more you learn, the more you want to learn. Soon she came across the globally recognized certifications conducted by the Yoga Certification Board. Confident in her previous preparation she decided to pursue **Level 3- Yoga Teacher and Evaluator.** The aptly structured syllabus of the YCB course introduced her to the great knowledge of Veda and Upanishads. Post clearing the YCB Level 3, she decided to further her learning with an **MSc (Yoga)** and an **MSc (Vedanta).**

About The Author

Apart from **Complete Guidebook For YCB Level 2 Yoga TTC**, she has also authored compiled study material for **Complete Guidebook For YCB Level 1 Yoga TTC** in English as well as in Hindi, **Complete Guidebook For YCB Level 3 Yoga TTC,** and **a Question bank with over 1500 Multiple choice questions for YCB exams.**

Nidhi has put her heart and soul into compiling this guidebook as she understands the difficulties faced by the students in finding the right kind of study material. It's our heartfelt wish that our learners find this useful. We wish all the very best to the aspirants, may you all be full, healthy, and wise!

Nidhi can be reached @ yogafitness.nidhi@gmail.com

ABOUT AYUSHMAN YOG

*A*yushman Yog is an exceptional online platform dedicated to preparing students for the YCB Yoga TTC. With our specialized curriculum and experienced instructors, we offer comprehensive training at an affordable fee, making it accessible to aspiring Yoga teachers from all backgrounds. By focusing on the specific requirements of the YCB syllabus, Ayushman Yog ensures that students receive targeted guidance and resources to excel in their exams and embark on a fulfilling journey as certified Yoga Teachers. Visit our website **www.ayushmanyog.com** to explore our offerings, connect with experienced instructors, and embark on a transformative journey towards becoming a Certified Yoga Teacher.

INTRODUCTION

*I*ntroducing the groundbreaking first-of-its-kind, **"The Complete Guidebook for Level 2- 400 Hrs. Yoga TTC"**.

This Yoga Teachers Training Exam is conducted by the Yoga Certification Board (A body that functions under the Ayush Ministry). Clearing the exam earns you the prestigious title of **Yoga Wellness Instructor** and enables you to work as a government-certified Yoga Professional worldwide.

Earlier, Yoga aspirants struggled to study from many different resources to prepare for this exam, as there was no single book that comprehensively covered the syllabus for this exam.

This comprehensive guidebook revolutionizes the field of Yoga Teacher Training by providing a single resource that covers the **entire syllabus** of the course. From the fundamentals of Asanas, Anatomy, and Physiology to a wide horizon of Philosophy, Patanjali Yoga Sutra, Various Hatha Texts, Deep understanding of Human psychology, this guidebook is your ultimate companion in mastering the art and science of Yoga. Furthermore, it goes above and beyond by including a compilation of 450 multiple-choice questions, enabling you to test your knowledge and preparation for becoming a skilled **Yoga Wellness Instructor**.

Introduction

To make the **most of this comprehensive guidebook**, download the syllabus pdf of YCB Level 2 from the website of the Yoga Certification Board. https://yogacertificationboard.nic.in/, then start by familiarizing yourself with the table of contents, which outlines the syllabus in a structured manner. Dive into each section, reading and absorbing the knowledge provided. Use the 450 MCQs strategically as self-assessment tools to gauge your understanding and identify areas for further study.

Follow Unit 4 to understand the practices and ensure an everyday practice routine to enhance the experiential dimension of yoga abhyas.

Approach this book as a roadmap for your journey toward becoming a skilled **Yoga Wellness Instructor**, and let it be your trusted companion every step of the way.

Prepare to embark on a transformative journey towards becoming a confident, knowledgeable, and proficient Yoga professional.

ABOUT THE YCB LEVEL – 2, 400 HRS. YOGA TTC EXAM

When you feel prepared to take the yoga certification exams, you can book them on the website of the Yoga Certification Board. The exams consist of two parts: one is multiple choice questions, and the other is a demonstration. Both exams can be taken online, and the process is explained in detail on the board's website. You are required to score 70% in both exams, post which you will receive the certificate with the title **"Yoga Wellness Instructor".** This is one of the most prestigious certificates in the Yoga community and is valid internationally.

MCQ exam- In the online setting, this exam happens through a Live monitoring process. You will not be able to open any other tabs on the computer, also you will be requested to not make much movements. This is to ensure the authenticity of the exam. There is no negative marking.

Practical- A panel of 4-5 examiners will be taking this exam. The duration would be 20-30 minutes. All the demonstrations will be based on Unit 4 of the syllabus. Additionally, they will be asking you to recite the sutra (refer to chapter 2.4). You would also be asked to chant a prayer at the beginning of your exam and explain the meaning of it.

They may also ask you some of the important concepts of yoga philosophy such as Panchakosha theory, Panch Prana, the meaning of Yoga, Ashtanga yoga, etc.

This book gives you comprehensive information about the complete syllabus. Ensure that you prepare well and keep testing your knowledge through the MCQs.

All The Best

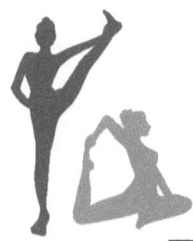

UNIT 1

INTRODUCTION TO YOGA AND YOGIC PRACTICES

1.1 Yoga: Etymology, Definition, Aim, Objectives

Etymology - The word etymology means the study and understanding of the origin/ source of the word. In Hindi, it's called- **Vyutpatti Shastra.**

So when we talk about the etymology of the word yoga, we are trying to understand how the word originated. Where is it sourced from? What might be the Sanskrit root?

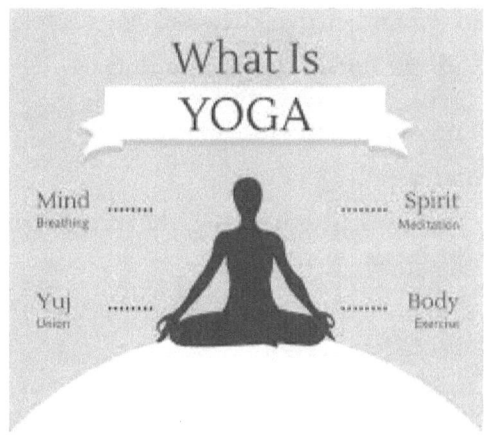

The Sanskrit word "yoga" is derived from the root word "Yuj", which means to yoke, harness, or join. It is understood that the 6th-century grammarian **Panini** has derived the term **Yoga** from either of the two roots

- **Yujir Yog** or
- **Yuj**

Based on the meaning of the root word **Yuj- Union**, yoga is commonly understood to mean union.

- **Yuj Samyoga** - To unite.

Now, when we say "**To unite or the union**" " the question comes, "the union of what?" The answer to this is- **the union of the individual self with the supreme self.**

However, that's not the only meaning of the word Yoga. There are 2 more meanings that come when using the same root "Yuj". Which are-

- **Yuj Samadhau** - To integrate
- **Yuj Samymane** - To restrain

We should also remember that the word yoga is referred to as the **Sadhya and Sadhna both.** This means that -

- Yoga is the end objective (Sadhya) - the union of the individual self and supreme self,
- As well as the Sadhna, meaning the **means, method, and technique** to achieve that union.

Definition of yoga as per different texts-

Different teachers have given different definitions of Yoga as per their perspectives, and understanding. For example

Sage Patanjali, who is also referred to as the **Father of Yoga** defines Yoga as the control of the fluctuation of the mind. Now before we discuss the definition given by him, Let's talk about him a little, and let's also read a legend about his birth.

First, Why is he called the Father of Yoga?

We should understand that yogic knowledge goes back to the **Vedas** and these are known to be the oldest scriptures in our culture. The first written record of Yogic knowledge is found in the Vedas. This also means that yogic knowledge was already prevalent in society in the verbal form before it was written because written records will always come later, at first the knowledge is always spread through word of mouth. We are talking about a time when **Guru-Shishya Parampara** was followed. Hence it is believed that everybody was aware of yogic practices and yogic knowledge.

But this wholesome knowledge was scattered.

Sage Patanjali was the first one, who gathered all this knowledge and structured it in the form of sutras, and presented it to the world in the form of **a book**. The book is famously known as **Patanjali Yoga Sutra**. This was the first structured representation of yogic science and due to this contribution, Patanjali is referred to as the Father of Yoga. The book contains 196 or some say 195 sutras. The difference is due to one sutra which many commentators found to have more of a repetitive meaning. Hence 195 or 196, both numbers are accepted.

> Sutra- One-line Sanskrit sentences that are connected.
>
> Adi Yogi- Don't get confused with Patanjali and Adi yogi, Adi yogi means the First Yogi who is Lord Shiva, Shiva gave the knowledge of yoga to the Saptarishi and Saptarishi then spread the knowledge across the world.

The Great Legend-

Once it happened that Adi yogi Shiva was doing **Tandava Nritya,** and the dance was so exquisite that lord Vishnu who was lying on **Shesha-Naga** started to vibrate to the rhythm of that Nritya. Lord Vishnu gets so absorbed in the rhythm that he starts to move with the rhythm, up to the extent that Shesha-Naga starts to feel discomfort as Lord Vishnu keeps moving.

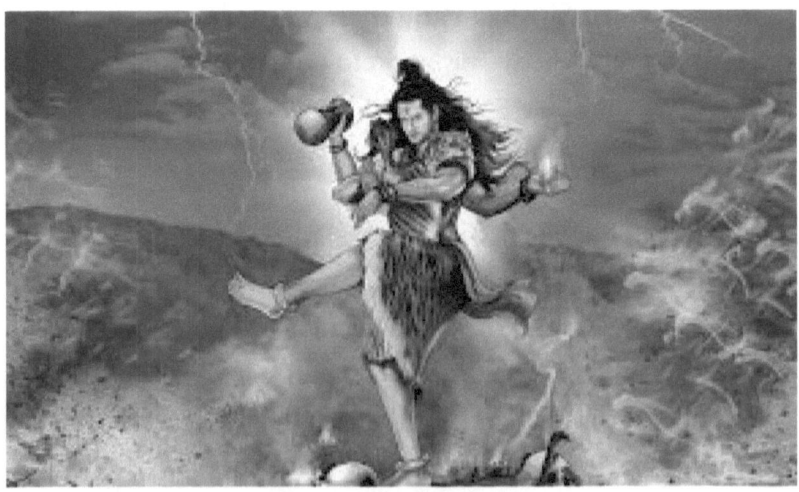

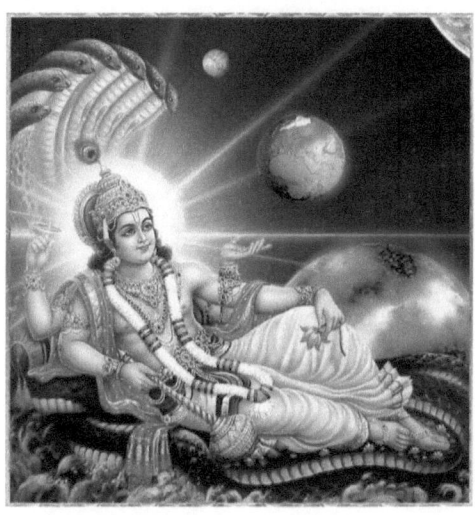

Then, when the Nritya ends, Lord Vishnu comes back to his senses and realizes the discomfort of Shesha-Naga. Shesha-Naga asks him what happened, Lord Vishnu then explains to him about Adi yogi, Tandava Nritya, Yoga, etc. Shesha-Naga becomes so overwhelmed that he said he wants to learn all of this knowledge. So he asks for a boon from lord Vishnu and Lord Vishnu says that soon enough Shesha-Naga will take birth on earth and will get opportunities to learn all this and more.

Sheshnaga gets very excited and he starts to meditate to know who is going to be his mother. Now, on earth, there was an ardent yogini named **Gunika.** She is a Brahmacharini and she wanted to give all of her knowledge to someone, but could not find the right disciple.

Once she was praying after taking bath in the river for a child and as soon as she opened her eyes she saw a small baby snake in her palms which were folded in Anjali mudra.

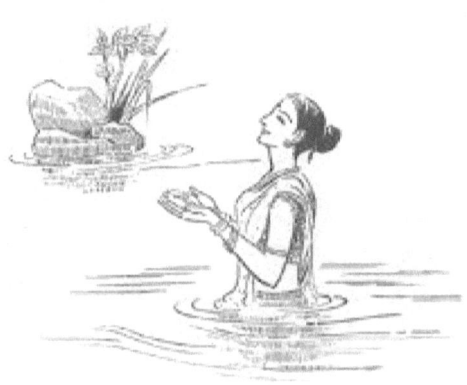

To her surprise that baby snake quickly transformed into a human baby. **Gunika** took it as a sign from the supreme and took the child as her son and used the incident to name him. **Pat means fallen, and Anjali- means the way her palms were folded. Hence Patanjali, meaning fallen into the palms.**

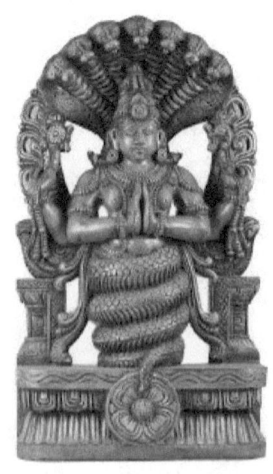

Interesting, isn't it?

Now coming back to the topic-

The definition of Yoga according to **Patanjali** is given in the 2nd sutra which is

- **Yoga-chitta-vritti-nirodhah ||PYS 1.2||**

<u>Meaning</u> - The complete cessation of fluctuation (Chitta-Vritti) of the mind is yoga.

Yoga has been explained in the Bhagwad Gita as well. Let's look at some of the very popular definitions.

2. **Bhagavad Gita-**

- **yoga-sthaḥ kuru karmāṇi sangam tyaktvā dhanañjaya,**

siddhy-asiddhyoḥ samo bhūtvā samatvaṁ yoga uchyate

||BG 2.48||

yoga-sthaḥ—being steadfast in Yog; **kuru**—perform; **karmāṇi**—duties; **Sangam**—attachment; **tyaktvā**—having abandoned; **dhanañjaya**—Arjun; **siddha-asiddhyoḥ**—in success and failure; **samaḥ**—equipoised; **bhūtvā**—becoming; **samatvaṁ**—equanimity; **yoga**—Yog; **uchyate**—is called

<u>Meaning</u> - Be steadfast in the performance of your duty, O Arjun, abandoning attachment to success and failure. Such equanimity is called Yog.

- **buddhi-yukto jahātīha ubhe sukṛita-duṣhkṛite**

tasmād yogāya yujyasva yogaḥ karmasu kauśhalam

||BG 2.50||

buddhi-yuktaḥ—endowed with wisdom; **jahātih**—get rid of; **iha**—in this life; **ubhe**—both; **sukṛita-duṣhkṛite**—good and bad deeds; **tasmāt**—therefore; **yogāya**—for Yog; **yujyasva**—strive for; **yogaḥ**—yog is; **karmasu kauśhalam**—the art of working skilfully.

<u>Meaning</u> - One who prudently practices the science of work without attachment can get rid of both good and bad reactions in this life itself. Therefore, strive for Yog, which is the art of working skilfully (in proper consciousness).

- yuktāhāra-vihārasya yukta-cheṣhṭasya karmasu

  yukta-svapnāv-abodhasya yogo bhavati duḥkha-hā

||BG 6.17||

yuktaḥ—moderate; **āhāra**—eating; **vihārasya**—recreation; **yukta cheṣhṭasya karmasu**—balanced in work; **yukta**—regulated; **Swapna-avabodhasya**—sleep and wakefulness; **yogaḥ**—Yog; **bhavati**—becomes; **duḥkha-hā**—the slayer of sorrows.

<u>Meaning</u> - But those who are temperate in eating and recreation, balanced in work, and regulated in sleep can mitigate all sorrows by practicing Yog.

- taṁ- vidyāt- duḥkha- samyoga- viyogaṁ- yoga- sañjñitam

  sa- niśhchayena- yoktavyo- yogo- nirviṇṇa- chetasā

||BG 6.23||

tam—that; **vidyāt**—you should know; **duḥkha-samyoga-viyogam**—state of severance from union with misery; **yoga-saṁjñitam**—is known as yog; **saḥ**—that; **niśhchayena**—resolutely; **yoktavyaḥ**—should be practiced; **yogaḥ**—yog; **anirviṇṇa-chetasā**—with an undeviating mind

<u>Meaning</u> - That state of severance from union with misery is known as Yog. This Yog should be resolutely practiced with determination free from pessimism.

3. Kathopnishad-

- Tam - yogam- iti- manyante- sthriam- indriyam- dharnam |

apramatt- stada- bhavati- yogo- hi- prabhva- apyayau ||

<u>Meaning</u> - The state when the senses are imprisoned in the mind, of this they say "it is Yoga". The man becomes very vigilant, for yoga is the birth of things and their endings. **"Stability of senses"** is considered Yoga.

Aim & Objective -

- The ultimate aim of Yoga is to set the individual free from the sufferings of life. As suggested in Ashtanga Yoga of Patanjali, the final goal (8th limb) of yoga is samadhi. In Hatha yoga also the eventual objective of Yoga is **samadhi.**

- However, it is important to understand that reaching the final goal involves a systematic plan of action. **This plan of action takes into consideration all aspects of human existence, i.e., physical health, the breathing process, health of internal organs, mental health, moral health, spiritual health, etc.**

The various stages/steps in Yoga practice prepare the body for higher spiritual sadhana.

- As intriguing as it sounds, one may still question one's willingness to walk on this path to achieve samadhi. And that's when one realizes the beauty of Yoga, **that even if one is not inclined towards the higher spiritual sadhanas, you can still take care of your body with it.** The Asana practice will ensure a healthy disease-free body, Pranayamas will help you get control of your breath and the mind, and cleansing practices (Kriyas) will clean the body from the inside.

Staying healthy is a global requirement, and yoga is the means to fulfill it.

Misconceptions- Misconceptions happen due to a lack of awareness. We need to educate our practitioners about the true meaning and nature of yoga. And we can only do that once we are aware of it. Some of the common misconceptions about Yoga can be -

- Yoga is physical exercise.
- To be able to do Yoga, one has to be in a certain shape or within a certain age group.
- Yoga should be avoided by expectant mothers.
- One should be flexible before starting a Yoga practice.
- It doesn't give a high-intensity exercise to the body; it is very slow.
- It is only for women.

1.2 Yoga: Its origin, history, and development

Historical evidence of the existence of yoga was seen in the pre-Vedic period (4500 - 2700 BC). We know that the first written reference to Yoga is mentioned in the Vedas. This means that yogic knowledge existed even before the Vedas. As we discussed in the last chapter, knowledge always exists in the verbal form first, and then the written record comes. So, we can say that yogic knowledge and practices definitely existed from the pre-Vedic **period.**

The main sources from which we get information about yoga practices and the related literature during this period are;

- Vedas (4)
- Upanishad (108)
- Smriti
- Teachings of Buddhism
- Teachings of Jainism
- Panini
- Ramayana
- Mahabharat
- Puranas (18) etc.

Now, let's understand how yogic practices have changed with time. To do this, let's divide the timeline into five periods.

1. Vedic Period
2. Pre-Classical Period
3. Classical Period
4. Post-Classical Period
5. Modern Period

1. The Vedic period-

This period is marked by the emergence of the Vedas. Vedas are the earliest written text in our culture. These are also known as Shruti. Shruti means that which is heard. It is said when the rishis used to go into deep meditation, they used to hear sounds. When they focused on these sounds, they became clearer, and Rishis realized those to be the mantra/hymns.

Rishis wrote down these mantras and the collection of such mantras is referred to as Vedas. The contribution was made by several rishis, male and female.

Also, understand that initially, there was just one book, and it was called **Rigveda**. Later on, the book was divided into 4 books, which then came to be known as 4 Vedas. There is not much known about how and when this division took place; however, when one reads the 4 Vedas, one can see that every Veda has a particular theme. Such as -

The Rig Veda - Consists of hymns that are used to praise divinity. The famous Gayatri Mantra comes from Rigveda

The Sama Veda - Has a lot of mantras from Rig Veda, but these are to be chanted melodiously.

The Yajur Veda - Contains the knowledge of rituals and yajnas.

The Atharva Veda - Contains the knowledge of science, ayurveda, economics, the code of everyday life, etc.

The Vedas are generally divided into two sections.

1. **Karma Kanda (Ritual Portion)**

2. **Jnana Kanda (Knowledge Portion)** - This part of Veda is also known as Upanishad / Vedanta. Upanishads talk about three subjects

1. Jeeva or the individual souls,
2. Jagat or the world and
3. Ishwara or the supreme

During this period, groups of Rishis practiced tapas by gathering around a fire (Havana Kunda) and making primordial sounds (Mantra). These Rishis realized the ultimate truth through their intense spiritual and meditative practices.

Mainly, three types of yoga practices were prevalent.

1. **Mantra Yoga** - Mantras were used as tools for the transformation of the mind. Disciples used to get mantras from their gurus.
2. **Prana Yoga** - Pranayama practices were used to control the Prana in the body.
3. **Dhyan Yoga** - Meditation practices were very common and meditation was suggested as the best tool for higher spiritual realizations.

> **Mantra** - A mantra is a sacred phrase or a syllable that, when chanted continuously with faith leads to spiritual realization, Such as Om Namah Shivaya, Om Namo Bhgawate Vasudevaya Namah, Om, lam, ram, kham, etc.

> **Prana** - Prana is the vital force in our body. It is known to be some element that keeps us alive as well as keeps the body functioning at its best. Prana cannot be misunderstood with mere oxygen. If oxygen were to be prana, then no one would be dead. In the coming chapters, we will study the prana and pranayama in detail.

2. Pre-Classical Period -(1500 – 1000 BC)

The Upanishad forms the main texts of this period. Along with that, another remarkable yoga scripture during this time is **Bhagavad Gita** which was composed around 500 BC. During this period, 4 paths of Yoga were taught. They are;

1. **Karma Yoga** – Yoga of perfect action
2. **Bhakti Yoga** – Yoga for perfect devotion
3. **Gyan Yoga** – Yoga of perfect knowledge
4. **Raja Yoga** – Yoga of willpower

3. Classical Period- (100 BC – 500 AD)

- The first systematic and coherent presentation of yoga was done by the **Sage Patanjali** in the classical period when he brought out the Patanjali Yoga Sutra. This work is generally believed to be dated between the 3rd and 6th BC or around 200 BCE - 200 CE.
- There is a total of **195 sutras** in PYS. (Some say 196, that is also true)
- **Ashtanga Yoga** is propounded in PYS.
- The earliest known Sanskrit commentary on the Sutras is **Yoga Bhashya** by sage Veda Vyasa in the 5th century.

Ashtanga Yoga-

1. **Yama** - Social restraints/observances or ethical values
2. **Niyama** - Personal observances, restraints
3. **Asanas** - Physical postures
4. **Pranayama** - Control of life force through breath control or regulation
5. **Pratyahara** - Sense withdrawal in preparation for meditation
6. **Dharana** - Concentration
7. **Dhyana** - Meditation
8. **Samadhi** - Spiritual absorption

4. Post-Classical Period- (500AD – 1300 AD)

- This period in yoga affirms the teachings of Vedanta, which states that there is ultimate unity in everything in the cosmos. **Adi-Shankaracharya** was Vedanta's most prominent teacher at that time.
- **Ramanujacharya and Madhavacharya** were the other distinguished figures during this period.
- The teachings of **Surdas, Tulsidas, and Meerabai** were great contributions during this period.
- The earlier eras saw yogis laying emphasis only on meditation and contemplation. Their goal was to shed the mortal coils and merge with the infinite. But during this period, yogis began to probe the hidden powers of the body and Tantra Yoga was developed. **Tantra Yoga was then foreseen to be misunderstood by the people and the mystic practices were removed from it, and what remained is called Hatha Yoga.**
- The Nath Yogis of the Hatha Yoga tradition such as **Matsyendranath** were given the utmost respect. He is

considered 2nd after Shiva (Adi yogi). **Gorakshanath** was his prime disciple.
- **Chaurangi Nath, Swatmaram-Suri, Gherand, and Shrinivas-Bhatt** were some of the great personalities who popularized Hatha Yoga during this period.

What are dualism and non-dualism?

These can be termed the 2 main concepts of Santana culture. To put it in the simplest way possible, one line of thought in our culture says that the supreme and the individual's soul are 2 different entities. The individual souls are part of the supreme. This concept is referred to as **Dualism or Dvaita Siddhant.**

Another line of thought says that the individual soul and the supreme are one. Every individual soul has a supreme nature, but this realization is veiled due to ignorance and the objective of humans is to realize this truth. This concept is referred to as **Non-Dualism or Advaita Siddhant.**

Adi Shankaracharya was one of the main teachers of this concept. The very popular Mahavakyas- Aham Brahmasmi means I am the Brahma, is in the context of non-dualism.

Now, think about these concepts and try to understand what you relate to. Remember, this is not a matter of one concept being inferior or superior to the other, Instead, look at it from the perspective of 2 different paths that have the same destination.

5. Modern Yoga- (1700 AD – now)

The popularity of Yoga, which we see today, is all because our modern teachers kept holding on to the practices. Of course, they introduced their own perspective, and different lineages were created, but it's because of this contribution only, we know Yoga as we do today. For example, who can forget the famous parliament of religion in 1893 where Swami Vivekananda spoke about this great Yogic Knowledge? This was a very significant event because those were the times of British rule and missionaries used to be sent to India for conversions as they didn't understand our ways of life and thought of it as inferior. That is when Swami Vivekanand famously showed the world **how India is and will always be the spiritual teacher of the world.**

- The modern age of yoga can be said to begin with the traveling of some renowned Yoga masters to the West. The most prominent among them is **Swami Vivekanand.**
- A landmark day of modern-day Yoga may be **1893** when the Parliament of Religions was held in Chicago, USA.
- After Swami Vivekanand, the next prominent figure in the West was **Paramahansa Yogananda**, who arrived in Boston (1920). His teachings are called **Yogada Teachings.**
- Paul Brunton, a former journalist, editor, and author of the famous book A Search in Secret India, introduced Ramana Maharshi to Western seekers.
- From the early 1930s till his death in 1986, **Jiddu Krishna Murti attracted Western** minds with his philosophical thoughts. He expounded the wisdom of **Gyan Yoga.**

- In the mid-1960s **Maharishi Mahesh Yogi** introduced **transcendental meditation** to the west. He was associated with The Beatles.
- In 1965, **Shrila Prabhupadaa** came to the USA and founded the International Society for Krishna Consciousness **(ISKON)**. He spread a movement based on Bhakti Yoga.
- One of the most prominent yoga gurus was **Swami Sivananda Saraswati**. He served as a doctor in Malaysia and opened yoga centers in Europe and America. His famous disciple was **Swami Vishnu-Devananda**, who wrote the book Complete Illustrated Book of Yoga.
- **Rajneesh**, also known as Osho, was a widely popular guru in the 1970s and 1980s.
- The great **Shri Krishnamacharya** taught **Viniyog Hatha yoga**. His son, **Desikar,** and Desikar's brother-in-law, **BKS Iyengar** continued the tradition.
- In present times, several lineages are practiced such as Iyengar Yoga, Ashtanga Vinyasa Yoga, Isha Yoga, Upa Yoga, Hatha Yoga, Kriya Yoga, etc. But remember the objective of the practice, irrespective of the time has always been the union. **Which is Yoga, The union of the individual soul with the supreme soul.**

1.3 Brief Introduction to Samkhya and Yoga Darshana

The journey of understanding oneself often leads to questioning the reasons for one's own existence. Human minds have always tried to understand the nature and reason of life, death, the world, universe, cosmos, God, etc. These inquiries, many times lose direction, but sometimes, some of the brilliant intellects don't lose the objective, and their continuous analysis, calculations, and curiosity do yield results in terms of a philosophical perspective.

Though 'philosophy' means 'love of knowledge', the Indian systems went beyond the concept of knowledge. Our great teachers took this "inquiry" as a constant intellectual exercise that helped them get a clearer and deeper understanding of the meaning of life through intuitive perception,

That's how the name **Darshana** comes which means - seeing or experiencing.

The various Hindu philosophies can be classified into two schools

1. <u>The Astika school (The Orthodox school)</u> - The term "Astika" is derived from the Sanskrit word "Asti" which literally means "knowing that which exists". The Astika schools consider the Vedas as the authoritative and reliable source of knowledge. There are 6 schools of thought that come under Astika Darshan, These are collectively referred to as **Shad Darshan.**

- **Nyaya-** Mahrishi Gautama
- **Vaisheshika-** Maharishi Kanad
- **Samkhya-** Mahrishi Kapila
- **Yoga** - Mahrishi Patanjali
- **Purva Mimamsa-** Maharishi Jaimini
- **Uttar Mimamsa-** Mahrishi Veda Vyasa (Badarayana)

2. <u>The Nastika school (The heterodox school)</u> - The Nastika schools reject the Vedas as authoritative texts or sources of knowledge. The most popular Nastika schools are-

- **Buddhism** - Gautama Budha
- **Jainism**- Rishabhdeva was the first Tirthankara, Mahavir swami was the 24th Tirthankara
- **Charvak** - Mahrishi Brihaspati
- **Ajnani** - Sanjaya Belatthiputta
- **Ajivika**- Goshala Maskariputra also known as Gosala Makkhaliputta

> **The theory of cause and effect-** This theory talks about the basic question: Does the effect pre-exist in its material cause? Those who answer "No" are called Asatkaryavadins, while those who answer "yes" are called Satkaryavadins.
>
> **Asatkaryavadins-** This line of thought argues that effect is a new creation, a real beginning. The effect does not pre-exist in its material cause. Otherwise, there would be no sense in saying that it is produced or caused. For instance, If the pot already exists in the clay, then why should the potter exert himself in producing the pot out of the clay? Moreover, its production would be its repeated birth which is nonsense. Nyaya, Vaisheshika, Hinayana, Buddhism, Materialism, and some followers of Mimamsa believe in Asatkaryavadins i.e. The view that production is a new beginning.
>
> **Satkaryavadins-** The Satkaryavadins on the other hand believe that the effect is not a new creation but an explicit manifestation of that which was implicitly contained in its material cause. Such as- Oil pre-exists in the sesame seeds. Here another important question arises: Is the effect a real transformation or an unreal appearance of its cause? Those who believe that the effect is a real transformation of its cause are called **Parinamavadins** (parinama=real modification); while those who believe that it is an unreal appearance are called **Vivartavadins** (vivarta=unreal appearance). Sankhya, Yoga, and Ramanuja believe in Parinamavadins.

Samkhya Darshan-

Of all philosophical systems, Sankhya Darshan is considered to be the most ancient school of thought. In the Mahabharata, **it is said that there is no knowledge like Sankhya and no power like that of Yoga (Shanti Parva 316-2).**

- Sankhya is popularly referred to as **Uncompromising Dualism, Atheistic Realism, and Pluralistic Spiritualism.**
- **Dualistic** because it believes that the universe consists of two eternal and distinct realities- **Prakriti / Non-Self/ Material existence and Purusha / Self / Consciousness.**
- **Realistic** because it views that both matter (non-self) and spirit (self) are equally real; also, both are radically different from each other, as like, subject and object.
- **Pluralistic** because it believes the Purushas or souls are infinite in number. If the Purushas were one, all would become free if anyone attained Moksha. Samkhya says that the different souls are fundamentally identical in nature. There is no movement for the Purusha. It does not go anywhere when it attains freedom or release. Souls exist eternally separate from each other and from Prakriti. Each soul retains its individuality. It remains unchanged through all transmigrations. Each soul is a witness to the act of a separate creation, without taking part in the act.
- Prakriti remains unmanifested as long as the three Gunas - sattva, rajas & tamas - are in equilibrium. This equilibrium of the Gunas is disturbed when Prakriti comes into contact with consciousness or Purusha. The disequilibrium of the Gunas triggers an evolution that leads to the manifestation of the world from an unmanifested Prakriti.

- Prakriti is the source of everything in the world—all physical events and experiences, including self-consciousness, intellectual activity, and emotions.
- Everything in the universe (with the exception of Purusha) is composed of varying degrees of sattva, rajas, and tamas. Sattva is illuminating, Rajas is activating, and Tamas imposes limitations and restrictions. These three qualities are continually transforming and inseparable.
- Purusha ("Pure Consciousness") cannot create anything of its own accord. It is only when Purusha witnesses Prakriti that the world comes into being and things are presented to consciousness.
- At first, the union (Samyoga) of these two principles seems mutually beneficial: Purusha is given something to "see" and Prakriti gains the illumination of consciousness.
- But Samkhya enquires further about this and realizes that this **identification of Prakriti with the Purusha** is the reason for unhappiness in our lives. Purusha is of **Nirguna** quality, it is a mere witness (Sakshi) of the ever-occurring thoughts, emotions, changes, etc. But due to ignorance, when Prakriti starts to identify itself with Purusha, then "ego" starts to manifest, which leads to dual experiences such as pleasure/pain, happiness/sadness, etc.
- To eliminate this identification, Samkhya suggests acquiring Viveka, which means discriminating between Purusha and Prakriti through knowledge of the 25 tattvas.

Tattva- Tattvas are used to explain the structure and origin of the Universe. These are the basic concepts to understand the nature of the absolute, the souls, and the universe. Tattvas account for the totality of the universe as a whole, and each human being. The 25 Tattvas of Samkhya philosophy are-

1. **Purusha-** (Transcendental Self)
2. **Prakriti-** (Primordial nature / Unmanifest),
3. **Mahat-** (Buddhi/intellect)
4. **Ahamkara-** (Ego/Consciousness of self)
5. **Manas** - (Mind)
6. **Jnanendriyan / Sense Organs (5)** - Nose (Ghrana), Eyes (Chaksu), Tongue (Rasana), Skin (Tvak), and Ears (Srotra).
7. **Karmendriyan / Motor Organs (5)** - Mouth (Vak), Hands (Pani), Legs (Padam), Anus (Payu), Genital (Upastha)
8. **Tanmatra / Subtle Elements (5)** - Sound (Shabda), Touch (Sparsha), Vision (Roopa), Taste (Rasa), Smell (Gandha)
9. **Mahabhutas / Gross Elements (5)** - Ether (Akasha), Air (Vayu), Fire (Agni), Water (Jala), Earth (Prithvi)

Pancha Mahabhutas	Tanmatra	Jnanendriyan	Associated Finger
Akash	Shabda	Ear	Middle finger
Vayu	Sparsha	Skin	Index finger
Agni	Roopa	Eye	Thumb
Jala	Rasa	Tongue	Little finger
Prithvi	Gandha	Nose	Ring finger

Samkhya considers **3 Pramana** to gain reliable knowledge-

1. **Pratyaksha (Perception)-** As per texts Pratyaksha Pramana can be of two types: **External and Internal**. External perception is described as that which arises from the interaction of five senses

and worldly objects, while Internal perception is described as that of inner sense, the mind

2. **Anumana (Inference)**- It is described as reaching a new conclusion and truth from one or more observations and previous truths by applying reason. For instance- Observing smoke and inferring that there must be fire.
3. **Sabda (Verbal testimony)**- This is described as relying on the word, or testimony of past or present reliable experts.

Relevance of Samkhya-

Though life is meant to be a joyous experience our attachments, likes, and dislikes turn it into sorrow and pain. With experience and age, one learns to relegate the mental and physical suffering and monotony of life to the background of our thoughts in the name of managing them but they lurk there infinitely till a slight trigger puts them in the forefront once again.

One realizes that it is just impossible to permanently get rid of these miseries of life, or stop the new ones from emerging incessantly. The remedies available to one in this world are inadequate and short-lived in their effect. Medicines and drugs can temporarily create relief from certain ailments but cannot guarantee the complete non-occurrence of suffering in the future. One can even get addicted to drugs. That is the reason one is compelled to find a permanent solution to these pains.

The moment one is born one's connection to the supreme consciousness is severed by the attachments which emerge due to contact with the material world. As one grows, one continues to entangle with the ever-intensifying web of material attachments, this web of entanglements keeps one away from realizing the divinity present within oneself. **Realizing this divinity within oneself, or the supreme consciousness is the only permanent solution to all miseries of human life.** Samkhya says that only when Jiva attains knowledge does Purusha get separated from Prakriti and become eternally pure, i.e., it attains Mukti (liberation) from Prakriti.

Yoga Darshan-

Patanjali is called the father of yoga as he is the first one to structure and compile yogic knowledge in the form of **195** sutras, called **Patanjali Yoga Sutra.**

Patanjali Yoga Sutra is divided into 4 chapters-

Samadhi Pada- 51 sutra, Sadhna Pada - 55 sutra, Vibhuti Pada - 55 Sutra, Kaivalya Pada - 34 Sutra

Patanjali defines yoga in the second sutra as

Yogas chitta vritti nirodhah ||1.2||

Meaning - Yoga is the stoppage of mental modification.

Patanjali expounds on **Ashtanga yoga** which is an eight limbs system to achieve the supreme potential of human beings and the ultimate experience of Raja Yoga.

Ashtanga Yoga is discussed in detail in Chapter 2.5

1.4 Life sketches and teachings of Yoga masters

(Maharishi Ramana, Shri Aurobindo, Swami Vivekananda, Swami Dayananda Saraswati)

Maharishi Raman-

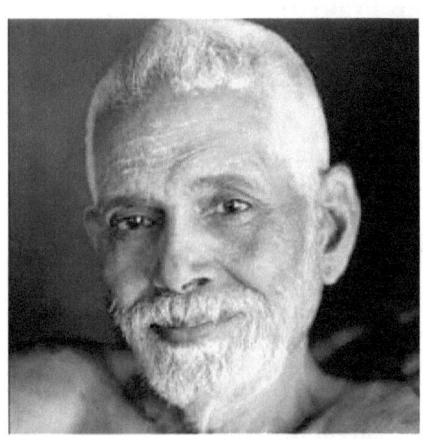

Birth and early years-

- Maharishi was born as **Venkatraman Iyer** to **Sundaram Iyer and Azhagammal** on **30th Dec 1879** in Tiruchuzhi village in Tamilnadu. His family was very religious. 2 of his family members had become sannyasins. He had a very good memory. He could recall information after hearing it once. He used to sleep very deeply, not waking from loud sounds, not even when his body was beaten by others.
- When he was about 12 years old, he experienced a spontaneous deep meditative state. In his biography "Sri Raman Vijayan" the experience is mentioned in his own words," **some incomplete practice from a past birth was clinging to me. I would be putting attention solely within, forgetting the**

body. Sometimes I would be sitting in one place, but when I regained normal consciousness and got up, I would notice that I was lying down in a different narrow space."

- When he was 11 he was sent to his uncle for further education. So that he can get a govt job. In Around 1895 (almost 16 years of age), One day he was reading the Tamil version of the very famous Kannada epic poem, **Prabhulingaleele**. By reading this he realized that Arunachal is a real mountain. He somehow knew about its existence but was overwhelmed to know that it really existed.

Spiritual awakening-

- One day when he was alone in his room he was suddenly gripped by an intense fear of death. In the following few minutes, he went through a simulated death experience during which he realized that his real nature was Imperishable and that it was unrelated to the body, mind, or personality. Many spiritual people have reported such experiences but they are almost invariably temporary. In Venkatraman's case, the experience was permanent and irreversible. From that experience onwards his consciousness of being an individual person ceases to exist and it never functioned in him again.

- He told no one about this experience and for 6 weeks he kept up the appearance of being an ordinary schoolboy. However, he found it increasingly difficult to maintain, and at the end of the 6 weeks, he abandoned his family and went directly to the holy mountain of Arunachal.

- His love for the mountain was so great that from the day he arrived in 1896 until his death in 1950, he could never be persuaded to go more than two miles away from its base.
- After a few years, his inner awareness began to manifest as an outer spiritual radiance and many people started following him. Although he remained **silent** most of the time, he did teach his followers.
- His earliest followers started calling him Mahrishi Raman; a contraction of his name Venkatraman.

Teachings-

- **The self** - He defined that the real self or real 'I' is, not an experience of individuality, but a non-personal, all-inclusive awareness.
- **God** - He maintained that the universe is sustained by the power of the self. He said that God is not a personal entity, he is a formless being that sustains the universe.
- **Jnana** - the experience of self is called jnana or knowledge. Jnana is a direct and knowing awareness of the one reality in which subjects and objects cease to exist.
- **Silence** - The inner silence is self-surrender. And that is living without the sense of ego. Solitude is in the mind of humanity. Silence is ever speaking; it is the perennial flow of "language". It is interrupted by speaking; for words obstruct this mute language. Silence is permanent and benefits the whole of humanity.

Last Days-

- In 1948 a cancerous lump was found on his arm, which was removed but soon after another growth appeared. A complete amputation of the arm was required but Mahrishi refused
- When his followers begged him to cure himself he calmly replied, "why are you so attached to this body, let it go. And where can I go? I am here".
- On 14th April 1960, he breathed his last at the same time a shooting star was seen.

Swami Vivekananda-

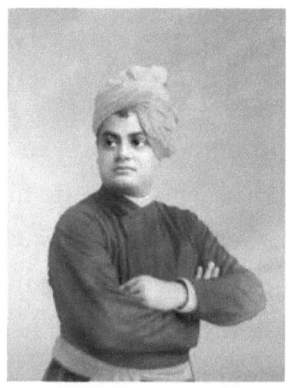

Birth and early years-

- On **12 January 1863**, a child was born in the famous Datta family to **Vishwanath Datta and Bhuvneshvari Devi**. The couple lovingly named the child **Narendranath Datta.**
- Narendra's father was a very learned man with proficiency in English and Persian. He was an attorney at law in the high court of Calcutta. His mother was exceptionally intelligent, and

spiritual and noted for her unusual memory. His grandfather Durga Charan Datta was well-versed in Persian and Sanskrit but at the age of 25, he renounced worldly life and became a monk.

- His mother, **Bhuvneshvari Devi** had a great influence on the formation of his character.
- He would have a peculiar experience when he would try to go to sleep. As soon as he closed his eyes there appeared between his eyebrows a wonderful spot of light of changing colors, which would expand and burst and bathe his whole body with a flood of white radiance. As the mind became preoccupied with this phenomenon, the body would fall asleep. As it was a regular occurrence with him, he thought this phenomenon was natural for everybody.
- At the age of 6, he was sent to a primary school, and soon he adopted some inappropriate words. So he was removed and then was homeschooled with a private tutor.
- He was always full of energy and disliked monotony. He used to organize an amateur theatrical company and presented plays in the worship hall of his home. Then he started a gymnasium in his home but one of his cousins broke his arm so it stopped. He then took lessons in fencing, lathi play, wrestling, rowing, and many other sports. When he got tired of this he showed magic lantern pictures in his home. When this bored him he got interested in cooking. And not to forget that he was always the leader of the group, never any less.
- He also grew very close to his father as he attracted the intellect of his son. He would hold long conversations with him on topics that demanded depth, precision, and soundness of the thought.

He is the one who planted the idea in Narendra that **education is a stimulus to thought and not a superimposition.**

Experiences and inquiries-

- By the age of 16, his interest in learning grew so much that he used to master 3 years of lessons in just 1 year. In his own words, "it so happened that I could understand an author without reading his book line by line. I could get the meaning by just reading the first and the last line of a paragraph. As this power developed, I found it unnecessary to read even the paragraphs, I could follow by reading only the first and last lines on a page. Further, when the author introduced discussion to explain a matter and it took him 4-5 or even more pages to clear the subject, I could grasp the whole trend of his argument by only reading the first few lines".
- As and when he started reading more and more his intellectual horizon also began to widen. Gradually his doubts and questioning took the form of an intellectual tempest that rages furiously and made him restless. At this time he came in contact with **Keshav Chandra sen, leader of Brahmo Samaj.** This samaj protested against orthodox Hinduism such as image worship, divine incarnation, and **the need for a Guru.** Vivekananda joined this samaj and for a time the intellectual atmosphere did satisfy him but gradually he started to realize that if God has to be realized then he is nowhere close to this goal.
- He started asking many leaders of different religious sects that, **"Have they seen God?"** and nowhere did he find the answer satisfactory to him.

- One day in college, his principal Hastie was taking a class on Wordsworth and found it difficult to explain the ecstasy of the poet to his students. Then he said that for visual proof of such an experience, one might go to **Dakshineswar to see Ramkrishna.**

Finding the Guru-

- Post this incident, one day Narendra decided to go meet Ramakrishna to find out about his direct God experience. On his first visit, he actually considered Shri Ramakrishna a madman as he was talking in such unusual ways.
- But then he went back again this time observing him carefully and he realized that there really is no strangeness in his behavior. From his words and ecstatic states, he concluded that Ramkrishna really is a genuine man of God. His answers are like **"God can be realized. One can see and talk to him as I am doing with you. But who cares to do so?"** Such simplicity, the sincerity in his voice, reached Vivekananda's curious mind. But he still was in conflict.
- He once again went to the temple after a month and this time a strange event took place. Ramkrishna invited him to sit next to him and then Ramkrishna touched him and he got unconscious of the external World. In his own words," the touch at once gave rise to a unique experience within me. With my eyes open I saw the walls and everything in the room whirl rapidly and vanish. I was about to merge into an all-encompassing mysterious void. I started crying, I was so frightened". As soon as Ramkrishna stroked his chest, the experience just vanished.

- This experience challenged all his beliefs and philosophical Intellect. He could not understand how someone with just one touch, could revolutionize the mind. Mesmerism, hypnotism, the possibility of having a weak mind, Narendra analyzed every possibility but he couldn't deny the experience.
- He decided to visit the third time, and this time he was all defensive against any influence on the part of Ramkrishna. But once again, the moment he touched him he again lost all outward consciousness and when he came to himself he found Shri Ramkrishna stroking his chest. He was now fully convinced of the extraordinary nature of that mighty power that was working through Ramkrishna and accepted him as his Guru.
- Narendra would open his preconditioned mind of not needing the guru, aversion towards idol worshipping, and many other beliefs, and Ramkrishna patiently answers his queries, over and over again.
- Sometimes, During the last days of Ramkrishna, Narendra was praying for a vision of absolute. And he unexpectedly received it during a meditation session. This he marks as a milestone in his spiritual sadhana.
- When Ramkrishna commissioned him with spiritual work for the world, he was reluctant at first because he wanted to stay immersed in this experience. But he agreed to his guru's wish eventually.

Narendra to Vivekananda-

- After the passing of his guru, he got this urge to travel, He wrote to one of his friends, "I am going away, but I shall never come back until I can burst on society like a bomb".
- One incident is really enlightening. Narendra had this interesting discussion with the Prince of Alwar, he said "I have no faith in idol worship. I can't worship wood, earth, stone, or metal, like other people." Swami ji then looked at a picture of the Maharaj hanging on the wall. He asked one of the courtiers whose picture is this? Diwan answered it is of the likeness of our maharaja. Swami ji asked diwan to spit on it. Everybody was terrified. Swami ji then said that it is just a picture, maharaja is not bodily present in it. What is the problem? He then turned to the maharaja and said it's not you but in one sense it is you. One glance at it brings you into their minds. Therefore they considered it spitting on it disrespectful to you. Similarly, idol worshipping is worshipping an emotion and not the object as such. Maharaj then said with folded hands that no one has thrown light on this subject in this manner.
- All of this wandering had great educational value for him. He came to Kanyakumari and sat in meditation for 3 days, during this meditation he saw the whole of India, her past, present, and future, her centuries of greatness, and also her centuries of degradation. He realizes that an empty stomach is no good for religion.
- His whole life from then onwards was dedicated to helping the poor in any way possible. He made the plan to travel to the West. His intention was to ask the West for the means to improve the material condition of India in exchange for

the gospel of Vedanta. He started to discuss this with various people and soon his intention to attend the parliament of religions took a definite shape.
- Around March/April 1893 the required funds were arranged and before leaving for America, in the court of Maharaj of Khetri, **he assumed the name of Vivekananda by** which he was to be known in the future.

Parliament of religion-

- The road to attending the parliament of religions was not easy. Upon reaching Chicago, he received the information that no one would be admitted as a delegate without proper reference, and the time for being so admitted had expired. He realized that he came too early. A great depression came over him. He asked for help through a friend in Madras and applied to an official religious society but the chief of the society gave him a very discouraging reply.
- Money was also getting low now. He now made a decision to move to Boston, which is cheaper than Chicago. And in the train from Vancouver, he made his first American friend, a lady from Massachusetts who was awestruck by his personality and illuminating talks gladly asked him to stay in her house. She introduced him to professor J.H. Wright, who was from the Greek dept. of Harvard University. The professor became so deeply impressed with him that he insisted that he should represent Hinduism in Parliament.
- The professor solved the problem of credentials and gave him a ticket to Chicago. Vivekananda rejoiced at this divine intervention. But the wait was still not over. He lost the address

of the committee. Nobody would help the colored man. Tired and helpless he passed the chilly night in a big empty box found in the railway freight yard. In the morning, he wandered from door to door for food only to meet with insults and rebuffs from the fashionable residents of the metropolis.
- On and on he went, finally exhausted he sat down quietly on the roadside, at this time, the door of a residence opposite to him opened and a regal-looking woman descended and asked him, " sir, are you a delegate to the parliament of religions?" and then Mrs. George W Hale took care of his journey to the parliament office.
- The day of the conference finally arrived and he joined the group of all Oriental delegates. He kept on passing his turn hour after hour to the end of the day and when the chairman insisted, he rose from his chair and bowed down to Saraswati. His face glowed like fire, his eyes surveyed the huge assembly before him and when he opened his lips his speech was like the tongue of flame. The entire assembly rose to their feet with deafening shouts of applause on his first few words, "**Sisters and Brothers of America**". Rest is history.

Teachings and work-

- "If there is ever to be a universal religion, it must be one which will have no location in place or time, which will be infinite. Which will recognize the divinity in every man and woman and whose whole scope, the whole force will be centered in aiding humanity to realize its own true nature."
- "Assimilation and not destruction."
- "Help and not fight."

- "Awake, arise, and stop not until the goal has been achieved."
- After coming back to India, he established the **Ramakrishna Mission Association**. He translated many Upanishads into simple language for the common people to understand.
- Many Westerners became his disciples and participated in his work of helping the poor.

Last Days-

- During 1901 and 1902 he came back to Belur math and lived a simple life there. It appeared that he is now waiting for a certain day to which he would throw off the bondage of the body.
- Friday the 04th July 1902, after having a routine day, in the evening he went into his room and stayed in meditation for an hour then he laid himself on his bed, an hour later he changed sides and took a deep breath, another long breath and then all was calm and still. There was no awakening to this world of Maya.

Swami Dayananda Saraswati-

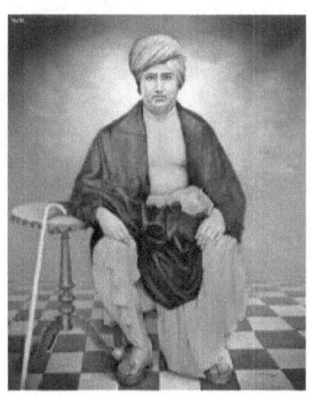

Birth and early years-

- He was born in a Brahmin Hindu family in Mul Nakshatra, to **Karshanji Lal ji Tiwari and Yashoda bai** on 12 February 1824. His parents named him **Mul Shankar**.
- His father was a follower of Shiva so he taught Mulshankar Shiva bhakti, fasting, and many other rituals.
- He usually kept fast and do Ratri Jagran on Mahashivratri. During one such fasting he noticed a rat eating the offering to Shivalinga and a thought occurred to him, why is this god not saving his food and his integrity from this tiny rat? The thought really troubled him.
- Another life-altering event was the death of his sister and uncle from cholera, and he again began to wonder about the role of God, the nature of life and death, etc.
- Not being able to get the answers and the pressure of marriage from his parents made him run away from his home at the age of 16.

The search for the Guru-

- For nearly 25 years he wandered in search of religious truth.
- He traveled to the Himalayas, spent his days in many forests, pilgrimages, and practice various styles of Yog, and then finally he met his Guru **Shri Virajanand Dandasheesha**.
- He was blind but his power to see was amazing. He believed that Hinduism had strayed from its historical roots and that many of its practice had become impure.
- Dayanand Saraswati then promised Virajanand that he would devote his life to restoring the rightful place of the Vedas in the Hindu faith.

Arya Samaj and Satyratha Prakash-

- He founded **Arya samaj** and gave 10 principles.
- **Satyarth Prakash;** Light of truth, which he wrote in 1875 is an eye-opener. Realizing the times when this book was written, was such a bold step. In this text, he clearly gives the name of scripture which he finds authentic as well as the ones which he finds fake. For yoga, he suggests reading Patanjali Yog Sutra only.
- He considered the authority of Vedas to be foremost and anything which is against the Vedas he holds as Adharma. Adharma was anything that did not hold true, was not just or fair, and was opposed to the teachings of the Veda.
- He explains very clearly the difference of opinions in Shaivism, Vaishnavism, Durga Mahatmaya, and almost all the different sects of Hinduism. He simply asked that in Shaivism Shiva Upasaka believes that the world is created by Shiva, Vaishnav believes it to be created by Vishnu, some by Durga, some by this, some by that. How can there be so many different opinions? Forget the other religions, how can there be so many different gods in one religion only?
- Questioning the authority of Puranas and many other scriptures, he said that people started writing scripture in the name of sacred sages so that it could be accepted widely. In Satyarth Prakash he mentions that Markandeya Purana and Shiv Purana were written during the time of Raja Bhoj by the name of Vyasa. When Raja Bhoj came to know about it he punished those Brahmans and clearly instructed everyone that write the scriptures by their name. This incident is mentioned in "Sanjivani" which is written by Raja Bhoj. This book

challenged the authority of many and many started considering him as the enemy.

Assassination-

- There were many assassinations attempts on his life due to his straightforward opinions which many considered controversial. In 1883, while staying at Maharaja of Jodhpur, he happened to see the maharaja with a dancer in a restroom. He advised the maharaja to forsake the girl and all the unethical acts and follow the dharma. The dancer named Nanhi Jaan decided to take revenge and conspired with his cook Jagannath. They gave Swami Dayanand a glass of poisonous milk which made Swami ji very sick. He was bedridden with excruciating pain. Seeing his condition the cook, Jagannath overwhelmed with guilt told him the truth, Swami ji forgave him and told him to flee the kingdom before the truth was found by the maharaja's men.
- On 30th October 1883, on the day of Diwali, he breathed his last chanting mantras.

Shri Aurobindo Swami-

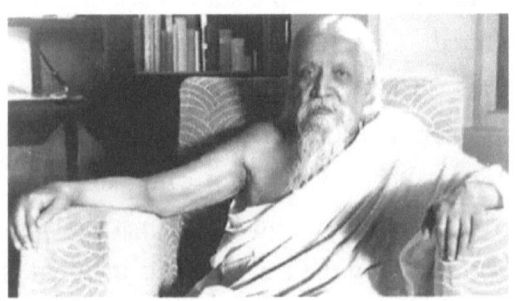

Birth and early years-

- Sri Aurobindo was born in Calcutta on **15 August 1872 to Krishna Dhun Ghose and Swarnalata Devi.** His father was a renowned surgeon.
- Young Aurobindo was brought up speaking English but used the local language to communicate with servants. Although his family was Bengali, his father believed British culture to be superior. He and his two elder siblings were sent to the English-speaking Loreto House boarding school in Darjeeling, in part to improve their language skills and in part to distance them from their mother, who had developed a mental illness soon after the birth of her first child.
- Darjeeling was a center of Anglo-Indians in India and the school was run by Irish nuns, through which the boys would have been exposed to Christian religious teachings and symbolism.
- In 1879, at the age of seven, he was taken with his two elder brothers to England for education and lived and studied there for fourteen years.
- He returned to India in 1893 and from 1893 to 1906 he worked in the Baroda Service, first in the Revenue Department and in secretariate work for the Maharaja, afterward as Professor of English and, finally, Vice-Principal in the Baroda College.
- During this time, he got interested in the Indian knowledge system and culture which he previously had no idea about. So, he learned Sanskrit and several modern Indian languages, assimilating the spirit of Indian civilization and its forms past and present.

- A great part of the last years of this period was spent on leave in silent political activity, for he was debarred from public action by his position at Baroda.

Political work-

- The outbreak of the agitation against the **Partition of Bengal** in 1905 gave him the opportunity to give up the Baroda Service and join openly in the political movement. He left Baroda in 1906 and went to Calcutta as Principal of the newly-founded Bengal National College.
- The political action of Sri Aurobindo covered eight years, from 1902 to 1910. During the first half of this period, he worked behind the scenes, preparing with other co-workers the beginnings of the Swadeshi movement.
- He was the first political leader in India to openly put forward, in his newspaper **Bande Mataram**, the idea of complete independence for the country. Prosecuted twice for sedition and once for conspiracy, and he was released each time for lack of evidence.
- In May 1908, he was arrested in the Alipore Conspiracy Case as implicated in the doings of the revolutionary group led by his brother Barindra; but no evidence of any value could be established against him and in this case, too he was acquitted. After a detention of one year as an undertrial prisoner in the Alipore Jail, he came out in May 1909. He spent this entire time in the practice of Yoga.

Spiritual Work-

- In February 1910, he withdrew to a secret retirement at Chandernagore and at the beginning of April sailed for Pondicherry in French India.
- Eventually, he cut off his connection with politics and went into complete retirement. During his stay at Pondicherry from 1910 onward he remained more and more exclusively devoted to his spiritual work and his sadhana.
- In 1914 after four years of secluded yoga, he began the publication of a philosophical monthly, the Arya. Most of his more important works, **The Life Divine, The Synthesis of Yoga, Essays on the Gita, and The Isha Upanishad,** appeared serially in the Arya.
- During his forty years in Pondicherry, he evolved a new method of spiritual practice, which he called **Integral Yoga**. Its aim is a spiritual realization that not only liberates man's consciousness but also transforms his nature.
- In 1926, with the help of his spiritual collaborator, his mother, he founded the Sri Aurobindo Ashram.

Last Days-

- Sri Aurobindo left his body on 5 December 1950.

1.5 Principles of Yoga

It is advised that Practitioners should follow some general principles of practicing yoga-

Before

- The place of practice should be cleaned. Yoga should be performed in a quiet and calm atmosphere.
- Yogic practices should be performed on an empty/light stomach. It's mostly because, on a heavy stomach, one would not be able to twist/bend comfortably. If you have just eaten, the internal organs especially the stomach will be engaged in digesting the food while feeling the pressure of the twisting / turning of asanas. The practitioner would not be able to utilize the practice time effectively.
- The bladder and bowels should be emptied.
- A mat, durry, or a folded blanket should be used. Don't practice on uneven surfaces.
- Light and comfortable (preferably cotton) clothes should be worn. Wear a shirt / T-shirt that won't come off while you perform an inverted posture or backbends.

Remember this sentence about the Prana, "Prana ensures the optimum functioning of the body". Let's understand how- Well this prana shakti actively does the healing work along with being responsible for digesting the food. However, it can only do one thing effectively at one time. So if you eat a heavy meal, the prana shakti would be engaged in digestion during the practice. Whereas if you are on a lighter stomach or empty stomach then the prana reservoir would be boosted and the healing will happen faster.

Now we agree that Yoga is an experimental science, so try putting this theory to use and see for yourself. Try practicing on an empty stomach for 21 days, then on a full stomach for 21 days, and then on a lighter stomach, and assess the results by yourself.

Remember that a good yoga teacher is a practitioner for life. So if you experience these by yourself only then you will be able to advise your practitioners with confidence and not sound bookish.

During-

- Practice sessions should start with a prayer. It is encouraged to chant a mantra but even Om chanting is sufficient.
- Breath awareness should always be maintained. Chest expansion and contraction should be specially emphasized.
- While releasing the posture, always release the way you went into the posture **(Last In, First Out).** This way, there would never be any chance of injury.

- Kumbhakas (Breath retention) should always be done with attention. Sometimes people tend to hold their breath while doing any advanced asana or while trying to hold the posture for a longer duration. This needs to be avoided. It is very important to continue breathing unless otherwise instructed.
- It's also important to understand that mastering a particular posture or mudra or Bandha, takes time. Staying patient with the practice is a secret that one should learn as early as possible.
- Contraindications of any asana/mudra/bandha/pranayama should always be followed.

After

- Don't shower immediately after practice. Give the body time to cool down on its own. Wait for a minimum of 15-30 minutes before taking a shower.
- Immediately eating after the practice is not advised, maintain at least 45- 60 minutes before eating.
- Always end the asana practice with a relaxation asana such as Shavasana, Makarasana, Balasana, etc. Shavasana is the most preferable one.
- Always end the class with Shanti-path/mediation. Be grateful for the opportunity to be able to practice that day.

Yoga Practices for Healthy Living-

- The science of yoga has numerous practical techniques as well as advice for a proper lifestyle to attain and maintain health and well-being.
- In the **Ashtanga yoga of Patanjali**, Bahiranga practices such as **Yama, Niyama, Asana, and Pranayama** help in producing

physical health, while Antaranga yoga practices of **Pratyahara, Dharna, and Dhyana** will produce mental health.
- Social behavior is first optimized through an understanding and control of the lower animal nature **(Pancha Yama)** and the development and enhancement of the higher human nature **(Pancha Niyama)**.
- The body is then strengthened, disciplined, purified, sensitized, lightened, energized, and made obedient to the higher will through **Asana.**
- Universal Pranic energy that flows through the body-mind-emotions-spirit continuum is intensified and controlled through **Pranayama** using breath control as a method to attain the controlled expression of vital cosmic energy.
- The externally oriented senses are explored, refined, sharpened, and made acute until the individual can detach themselves from sensory impressions at will through **Pratyahara.**
- The restless mind is then cleansed, focused, and strengthened through **Dharna.**
- If these six steps are thoroughly understood and practiced then the seventh step, **Dhyana / Meditation** is possible.
- Intense meditation produces **samadhi** or the ecstatic feeling of Union, and oneness with the universe. This is the perfect state of integration or harmonious health.
- **Hatha yoga** offers ways to clean the internal organs **(Shat Kriyas)** and the physical postures **(Asana)** to strengthen the muscles and joints.
- Then it moves to even subtler systems of **Nadi** and also offers ways to cleanse and balance the Nadi **(Pranayama)**.
- Then it gives ways to control and channel the energy/prana shakti at designated places in the body **(Mudras & Bandhas)**.

- Once all this is mastered, one can move to the deeper practice of gathering within and listening to oneself **(Meditation)**.
- Yoga also emphasizes the need for a healthy, nourishing diet that has an adequate intake of fresh water along with a well-balanced intake of fresh food, green salad, sprouts, unrefined cereals, and fresh fruits.

General Benefits-

Yoga practices offer numerous benefits. The only way to find out is "to practice". Some of the common benefits can be -

- Regular practice improves flexibility.
- It gives deep relaxation at the muscular level.
- It slows down the breath and maintains balance at the pranic level.
- It strengthens creativity and willpower at a mental level.
- It sharpens the intellect and calms the mind down at the intellectual level.
- It enhances happiness in life and equipoise at the emotional level.
- It manifests the inherent divinity in humans in all aspects of their life.

1.6 Principles and Practices of Jnana Yoga

Jnana Yoga is the path of intuitive philosophical searching. In Jnana yoga, the mind is used to inquire into its own nature. The fundamental goal of Jnana yoga is to become liberated from the illusionary world of Maya (self-limiting thoughts and perceptions) and to achieve the union of the **individual Self (Atman)** with the **supreme self (Brahman).**

This is achieved by steadfastly practicing the mental techniques of **contemplation and meditation.** Jnana Yoga utilizes a one-pointed meditation on a single question of self-inquiry to remove the veils of illusion created by the preconditioned mind, concepts, world views, and perceptions.

This practice allows one to realize the temporary and illusionary nature of **Maya** and to see the oneness of all things. It is the path of self-realization through discriminating the real from the unreal. The three principles of jnana Yoga practice are -
- **Sravana** - Listening or absorbing the instructions,
- **Manan** - Reflection or contemplation involving reasoning and arriving at intellectual conviction.
- **Nididhyasana** - Repeated meditation on convictions/ accepted truths.

Sadhana Chatushtaya - Sadhana Chatushtaya refers to the 4 attributes which help the Jnana Yogi to stay true to their path. Sadhana Chatushtaya helps in the preparation of intellect, emotion, and will. In other words, these are the qualities and qualifications required for success in the study of Vedanta.

1. **Viveka** - Discrimination between real and unreal
2. **Vairagya** - Detachment from the fruits of actions
3. **Shad Sampat** (Six Attributes)- **Sama** (to control the mind/calmness), **Dama** (to control the senses/self-control), **Uparati** (self-withdrawal/to withdraw the senses), **Titiksha** (Endurance, patience), **Shraddha** (Faith), and **Samadhan** (not losing sight of the goal)

4. **Mumukshutva** – Yearning for freedom.

Sapta Bhumika- There are 7 stages a yogi goes through while on the path of Jnana Yoga. This concept is explained **in Yoga Vashishtha.**

1. **Subheccha (good desire)** - To begin with, one should strive to develop a focus on the deep study of various Sanskrit texts with faith and respect. The practitioner should try to associate with the wise. He/she should also build the habit of performing virtuous actions without any expectation of fruits. This is the stage of **Shubhechha or good desire**. This stage will gradually strengthen the discrimination faculty in the practitioner's mind. Practitioners will develop detachment toward sensual objects.

2. **Vicharana (Philosophical inquiry)** - The second stage involves questioning, contemplation, and reflection on the principles of non-dualism. It is the stage of constant Atma Vichara (self-inquiry).

3. **Tanumanasi (Subtlety of mind/Bringing the focus to one object/Tenuous mind)** - This third stage is achieved when one understands all the necessary knowledge. In this step, the mind **"becomes thin like a thread" as** one lets go of all external stimuli to focus all of the attention inwards. The practitioner gets free from all of the attractions. This stage is also called **Asanga Bhavana.**

   Swami Sivananda explains the importance of this stage saying that If anyone dies in the third stage, he will remain in heaven for a long time and will reincarnate on earth again as a Jnani.

The above three stages can be included under the Jagrat Avastha (Waking Stage)

4. **Satwapatti (Attainment of Light / Self-Realization)** - In the fourth stage, the world appears like a dream and the karma begins to dissolve. A yogi will view all things in the universe equally in this stage. All the vasanas (desires) will get destroyed to the root.
   This can be included under the Svapna state.
5. **Asamsakti (Inner Detachment)** - In this stage, one becomes detached and selfless and will experience deep states of bliss. One will feel no difference between waking and dream states. This is the **Jivanmukti stage** in which there is the experience of **Ananda Swaroopa** (the Eternal Bliss of Brahman).

This will come under Sushupti.

6. **Padartha Bhavana (Spiritual Vision / Non-perception of objects)** - In the sixth stage, one begins to see the truth and understand the nature of **Brahman (Ultimate Reality).**
7. **Turiya (Supreme Freedom)** - During the final stage, one is united in super consciousness. All the Gunas disappear. This stage is above the reach of mind and speech. Moksha is attained in this stage.

1.7 Principles and Practices of Bhakti Yoga

Bhakti yoga is a path of unconditional love toward God. This is yoga for devotees. Bhakti yoga doesn't tell you where to direct that devotion or the specific methods by which you should do it. It is left to the devotee's personal preference. This path is famously taught by Shri Krishna to Arjun as mentioned in Bhagavad Gita.

Bhakti Yoga is considered to be **the easiest** and the most certain way of liberation in this Kali-Yuga.

As per the Bhagavad Gita, there are 4 types of Devotees of bhaktas- **Arta (The distressed), Artharthee (The desire for wealth), Jigyasu (The inquisitive), Gyani (Who is in search of knowledge of absolute).**

There is another very popular text called **Narada Bhakti sutra,** which is a collection of 84 sutras. This text is said to be written by Devarishi Narada himself. This text talks about developing selfless love toward God. The very famous concept of **Navavidha Bhakti** comes from **Narada Bhakti Sutra-**

Navavidha bhakti is a 9 limbs practice, of bhakti Yoga. These Limbs are- **Shravanam** (Hearing), **Keerthanam** (Chanting), **Smaranam** (Remembering), **Pada Sevanam** (Service), **Archanam** (Worshipping), **Vandanam** (Saluting), **Dassyam** (Being a servant), **Sakhyam** (Friendship), and **Atma Nivedanam** (Total surrender)

1.8 Principles and Practices of Karma Yoga

This is the path of action. This path is primarily chosen by those who are of an outgoing or action-oriented nature. Karma Yoga is one of the central teachings of the Bhagwad Gita. The concept is mentioned in Bhagwad Gita as chapter titled **Karma Yoga (The Yog of Action)**.

- Shri Krishan explains to Arjun that nobody can remain without action, even for a moment. Bound by their inherent modes of nature, all beings are always engaged in some work. Those who continue to work diligently to fulfill their responsibilities

externally, but internally are unattached to them are considered Superior.
- Bhagwad Gita says that one should continuously practice detaching oneself from the fruit of action by surrendering the consequences completely to God. This way, one would learn to let go of the "ego". Simply put, the path of Karma yoga is to do your duty with utmost care and dedication without any **expectations and attachments to results**
- Bhagavad Gita says, "You have the right to perform the duties but you are not entitled to the fruits of your action" **(Nishkam karma).**
- It also clarifies that **"Never consider yourself to be the cause (Hetu) of the results of your activities and never be attached to not doing your duty."**
- It says that inaction should not be the way of humans. One should perform the prescribed duties since action is superior to inaction. By not doing any activity, even bodily maintenance will not be possible.

The text also explains different types of Karma. These are- **Shukla - Karma** (White / Good), **Krishna - Karma** (Black / Bad), and **Ashukla - Akrishna Karma** (Balanced)

1.9 Concept and principles of Sukshma Vyayama, Sthula Vyayama, Surya Namaskara, and their significance in Yoga Sadhana

Yogic Sukshma Vyayama (Micro Exercises)-

Sukshma Vyayama can be understood as a set of warm-up movements that prepare the body for further advanced sequences/

asanas. However, it is different from the other warm-up movements such as running, jumping, etc., due to the special attention given to Breathing and Concentration points..

Sukshma Vyayama was designed and propagated by Maharishi Kartikeya Maharaj of Himalaya. He then taught this to his disciple Dheerendra Brahmachari, who propagated this knowledge to the world. Yogic Sukshma Vyayama has 48 exercises (mostly Isolated movements) that cover all the joints from head to toe.

Sthula Vyayama (Macro exercises)-

Sthula Vyayama or Loosening exercises refer to the set of exercises that help loosen the different parts of the body. These are more strenuous than Sukshma Vyayama and mostly involve more than one joint (compound movements). There are a total of 5 exercises in Sthula Vyayama. These are- - Hrid Gati, Sarvang Pushti, Rekha Gati, Utkurdan, Urdhva Gati.

Benefits - Sukshma and Sthula Vyayama play a very important role in asana practice as perfect warm-up movements before the Surya Namaskar or any other sequence.

Doing these movements reduces the chance of getting an injury.

This Vyayama works as a successful aid in injury rehabilitation and therapeutic yoga.

Senior practitioners, obese people, or any practitioner who cannot follow through with Surya namaskar / any other sequence, can greatly benefit from Sukshma Vyayama.

Surya Namaskar

Surya Namaskar is a **sequence of 12 asanas**. What makes it different from any other asana sequence is the Bhava involved in this practice. The Bhava (attitude) of gratitude towards lord Sun, the very source of life on this planet. In Surya namaskar, one uses the body as an instrument to pay respect to the lord sun, in 12 different ways. The sequence primarily engages the spinal column, wherein it arches and bends alternatively, repeatedly.

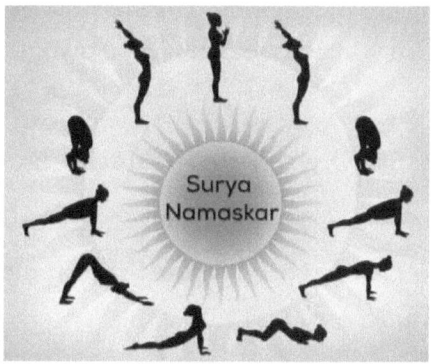

Every asana of Surya Namaskar has its respective mantra.

(For the demonstration exam it is important to memorize the mantra. You will be asked to perform Surya Namaskar with Mantra)

Pranamasana- Om Mitrye namah - Prostration to him who is affectionate to all.

Hastottanasana- Om Ravaye Namah - Prostration to him who is the cause of all changes.

Padahastasana- Om Suryaya Namah - Prostration to him who induces activity.

Ashva-Sanchalasana- Om Bhanve Namah - Prostration to him who diffuses light.

Parvatasana / Santolasana / Phalakasana- Om Khagaya Namah - Prostration to him who moves in the sky.

Ashtanga Namaskar / Sashtangasana- Om Pushne Namah- Prostration to him who nourishes all.

Bhujangasana- Om Hiranyagarbhaya Namah - Prostration to him who contains everything.

Parvatasana- Om Marichaye Namah - Prostration to him who possesses rays.

Asva-sanchalasana- Om Adityaya Namah - Prostration to him who is son of Aditi.

Padahastasana- Om Savitre Namah - Prostration to him who produces everything.

Hastottanasana- Om Arkaya Namah - Prostration to him who is fit to be worshipped.

Pranamasana- Om Bhaskaraya Namah - Prostration to him who is the cause of all lustre.

Different ways of practicing Surya Namaskara

- **With and Without Mantras**
- **With Antah-Kumbhak-**
    - In Pranamasana (first posture), Inhale and exhale.
    - With the next inhalation go to Hastottanasana and hold your breath inside (Antah-Kumbhak).

- o Finish the rest of the sequence while holding your breath in and exhale while coming back to Pranamasana.

- **With Bahya-Kumbhak-**
  - o In Pranamasana (first posture), Inhale and exhale and hold your breath out (Bahya Kumbhak).
  - o Finish the rest of the sequence while holding your breath out and inhaling while coming back to Hastottanasana.

Points to remember

- Every asana has its own breath pattern. It is important to stick to it.
- Aim for achieving perfection in all postures.
- Once the breath and movements have been mastered then learn to practice with breath control (Antah-Kumbhak / Bahya Kumbhak)
- Surya Namaskar works on all 5 parameters of fitness which are - Cardiovascular fitness, Strength, Stamina, Flexibility, and Body Balance.
- One can aim to do a number of repetitions of the whole sequence or increase the amount of time for holding every pose. Try to utilize this sequence as effectively as possible.
- Do not let go of the Bhava; Gratitude towards lord Sun.

Benefits

- Stretches, tones, and realigns the entire Musculo-Skeletal system.
- Improves mind and body coordination, and induces a feeling of composure within.

- The practice aims to energize and harmonize the physical structure. When combined with mantra chants and breath awareness the practitioner also engages the subtle body and deeper sections of the brain, which results in increased awareness and calmness.
- Ideal practice to incorporate in stress management, obesity management, and kid's Yoga.

Contraindication

- If one feels nauseated or giddy then lie down in Shavasana for some time. Always increase the number of rounds gradually.
- It should not be practiced by people suffering from acute cases of high blood pressure, hernia, or heart disease, and those who have had a recent stroke.

Someone with a back problem can practice it after consulting a yoga expert.
- It should not be practiced during fever and inflammation.
- It should also be avoided during menstruation.

1.10 Concept and principles of Shatkarma:

Meaning, Types, Principles and their Significance in Yoga Sadhana

Shatkarma

Shat - 6, Karma - Action.

The 6 cleansing methods suggested in Hatha Yoga for purifying internal organs are collectively referred to as Shatkarma.

We are going to do a comparative study of Shatkarma from **Hatha Yoga Pradipika (HYP) and Gheranda Samhita (GS)**. Both texts share two different perspectives about Shatkarma. Hatha Yoga Pradipika advised us to do these only in case of fat/mucus accumulation or any disease in the body whereas Gheranda Samhita kept these as a mandatory practice, even for healthy practitioners.

These are- **Dhauti, Basti, Neti, Trataka, Nauli and Kapalbhati.**

Benefits of Shatkarma

- When the body is purified, the chemical constituents are in balanced proportion and the brain functions are simultaneously influenced and altered. When the body is pure, the mind becomes stable, emotional reactions to external stimuli are altered and one will respond in a more relaxed and controlled manner.
- When Annamaya and Pranamaya koshas (Gross Koshas) are cleansed, there is no blockage between them and Manomaya Kosha (Subtle Kosha). Mind, body, and energy can work in unison, and that removes the barrier to Vijnanamaya Kosha.
- Shatkarma practice makes the Karmendriyan keen and Jnanendriyan more perceptive and sensitive.
- By the Shatkarma, one is freed from the excess of the doshas. Then pranayama is practiced and success is achieved without strain.

Dhauti - Stomach Cleansing:

Hatha Yoga Pradipika (HYP) mentions Vastra Dhauti.

- Make saline water and soak a strip of cloth, four fingers wide (7- 8cm), and 15 hand spans (one and a half meters or 22½ ft. approx.) in length.
- Now sit in Kagasana and slowly swallow the cloth as instructed by the guru. Once the 2/3rd of the cloth has been swallowed it can be left in the stomach for 5-20 mins. During this time one can stand up and do the Nauli also.
- Then, very slowly, take the cloth out of the mouth. One can see the residue of the stomach on the cloth. This is known as Vastra Dhauti.
- It is important to keep the cloth spread and not folded as you utilize it.
- The ideal time for this kriya is before sunrise.

> The reason to use saline water is to match the body's internal environment. Otherwise, if we use cold water or water with salt then the body will treat it as a foreign element and it would start to react. To avoid this, we use Saline water. To make 1 Ltr of saline water, mix 1 tsp of salt into 1 Ltr water and heat it then bring it to a lukewarm temperature.

Gheranda Samhita (GS) describes 4 types of Dhauti

Antar Dhauti	Danta Dhauti	Hrid Dhauti	Mool-Shodhan
Vatsara	Danta Shodhan	Vastra	
Varisara	Jivha Shodhan	Danda	

Vanisara	Karna Shodhan	Vaman	
Bahishkrit	Kapalrandhra Shodhan		

Antar Dhauti:

Vatsara- Vata means Air. The cleansing done with the element air is known as Vatsara. This is also known as Plavini.

Process- Draw the air slowly in through the mouth forming it like the beak of a crow (Kaki Mudra), move the abdomen, and then slowly expel the air through the anal route.

Varisara (Shankha-Prakshalana)- Vari means water. The cleansing done with the element water is known as Varisara. Varisara is also known as **Shankha Prakshalana**.

Shankha Prakshalana is of two types- Laghu Shankha Prakshalana and Deergha Shankha Prakshalana.

The difference between Laghu and Deergha Shankha Prakshalana is the amount of water that is used. In Laghu Shankha Prakshalana approximately 3-4 litres of water is used and in Deergha Shankha Prakshalana approximately 7-8 litres of water is used.

Process

- Prepare the saline water. Let's say we are doing Laghu Shakha Prakshalana so we will prepare 4ltrs of water,
- Now sit down and gulp down 1-2 Ltr of water so as to fill the stomach up to the throat. Then we have to push this water

down by moving the abdomen through different asanas and evacuate through lower passages. 5 asanas are to be done to achieve this - **Tadasana, Tiryak Tadasana, Kati Chakrasana, Tiryak Bhujangasana, and Udara-akarshana**

- Repeat these asanas multiple times until you get the urge to pass the motion. Then go to the toilet.
- Come back and again gulp down as much water as you can and repeat the process.
- This whole cycle is to be repeated until you finish the water or until absolutely clean water comes through the anus.

Bahishkrit (Rectal Cleaning) - This is an advanced practice and used to be done by ancient advanced Hatha yogis.

Process:

- Standing in navel-deep water, one should push out the Saktinadi (Rectum) and wash it with the hands to remove the filth. Then suck it all in again.
- The text says that this method of cleaning should be **kept a secret.** It is not easily available even to the gods.

> **Shankha means conch, and Prakshalana means cleansing.** This is a very interesting technique. The name comes from the conch cleansing itself. When you pour water into the conch, it comes out from the other way, similarly, the body is considered a conch, and one is supposed to drink water from the mouth, and then it should come out through the anal route. Now, water usually takes the route of the stomach, to the small intestine, to the kidney to the bladder.
>
> In Shankha Prakshalana kriya, this route gets altered so water then takes the route of the stomach, to the small intestine and then to the large intestine, and then to the anal cavity.
>
> This way the **entire GI tract gets cleaned**.

Danta Dhauti:

Danta- One should rub the root of the teeth with the extract of the Khadira plant (Acacia Catechu) or with clean earth until the impurity is removed.

Jihva- Putting the index finger, the middle finger, and the ring finger together into the throat, one should rub out the impurities and clean the root of the tongue slowly.

Karna Shodhan- One should rub the auditory canal by inserting the tip of the index finger into it. Through constant practice, an auditory sensation is experienced.

Kapal Randhra- Every day, after waking from sleep, after meals, and at the end of the day, one should rub the Bhalrandhra (the hindmost part of the roof of the mouth) with the right thumb.

Hrid Dhauti:

Vastra- The process of Vastra Dhauti is the same as mentioned in Hatha Yoga Pradipika. There is a slight change in the length of the cloth. As per Gherand Samhita, the cloth should be 4 fingers wide and 19-25 cubits in length.

Danda- In Danda Dhauti, a stick is used instead of cloth. Traditionally one should insert the stalk of plantain, turmeric, or cane into the gullet, move it there (up and down), and then slowly withdraw it out. These days this Dhauti is also done with a specially designed rubber tube.

Vaman- This is also known as Vyaghra Kriya. As per the Gherand Samhita, one has to drink water for 3-4 hours after eating. Then put the first two fingers down the throat and gently tickle the throat to stimulate the regurgitating reflex and vomit the remaining food from the stomach.

Mool Shodhan:

One should diligently clean the rectum with the stem of turmeric (plant), or the middle finger and water again and again.

Benefits Of Dhauti Kriya

- Cough, asthma, spleen disease, leprosy, and twenty kinds of diseases caused by excess mucus are destroyed through the effect of Dhauti karma.
- Dhauti Kriya (Antar and Hrid) cleans the entire digestive tract and respiratory tract. It removes excess and old bile, mucus, and toxins and restores the natural balance of the body's chemical composition.

- This kriya also helps remove infectious bacteria from the mouth, nose, eyes, ears, throat, stomach, intestine, and anus. The results are a reduction of excess fatty tissues, relief from flatulence, constipation, poor digestion, and loss of appetite.

Contraindication

- Antar Dhauti must not be practiced if you have stomach / intestinal ulcers, hernia, heart disease, and high BP.
- Dhauti shall (Antar and Hrid) also be avoided during the monthly period as the hormone balance may be affected.

In Hatharatnavali, Vaman Dhauti is described as Gajakarni (Elephant Stomach Cleansing). The process of both the kriyas are similar but the main difference is that in Gajakarni you are not required to drink water, whereas in Vyaghra kriya drinking water is required 3-4 hours after eating.

There is another form of Dhauti which is done on an empty stomach called **Kunjal Kriya.** This is usually the most practiced form of Dhauti these days. It can be done once a week then later on twice a month.

Process-

Make 2-3 liters of saline water. Sit in Kagasana and gulp down the water to fill the stomach up to the throat.

Then stand up, keep the feet together, and bend forward over the sink or bucket.

Place the left palm on the stomach and use the right index finger, middle finger, and ring finger to tickle the back of the throat to create a vomiting reflux.

The entire water would come out of the stomach along with the residue of the undigested food.

Half an hour after vomiting you should eat a liquid (not thick) preparation of sweet- boiled rice and milk or plain khichdi made in clarified butter (Desi Ghee). Avoid eating spicy food the day you perform Kunjal Kriya.

Basti (Yogic Enema)

HYP mentions Jala Basti.

- Sit navel-deep in water in Utkat asana, insert a tube into the anus, and contract the anus again and again. This cleaning with water is called Basti karma.
- To perform Basti, the practitioner first has to be adept in Uddiyana Bandha and Nauli.

GS mentions 2 types of Basti-

- **Jala Basti-** Same as mentioned above.
- **Sthal Basti / Shushka Basti-**
  - Lie down in Vipareeta Karani asana.
  - Now dilate and contract the anus by Ashvini Mudra.

Benefits:

- Enlargement of the glands and spleen and all diseases arising from excess air, bile, and mucus are eliminated from the body through the practice of Basti.
- By practicing Jala Basti, the appetite increases, the body glows, excess doshas are destroyed and the Dhatu, senses, and mind are purified.
- Basti completely washes the bowels and removes excess bacteria, old stool, threadworms, and heat from the lower intestines.
- Basti cures digestive disorders and is particularly useful for removing constipation, stimulating sluggish digestion, controlling nervous diarrhea, and strengthening the solar plexus.

Contraindication:

- This practice is contraindicated for people with rectal bleeding, ulcerative colitis, and colon cancer.
- Basti karma is also used as an **Ayurvedic panchakarma therapy** wherein herbal decoction mixed with honey, rock salt, etc. are administered en route like an enema. This is also called Asthapana Basti.
- Asthapana Basti should not be done if you have indigestion (Ajirna), Low Digestion (Alpa-Agni), are Very Weak (Ati-Durbalta), in the presence of hunger, thirst, tiredness, etc.

Neti (Nasal Cleansing / Irrigation)
HYP mentions Sutra Neti-

- Take a soft thread 4 mm wide and 36 cm long (approximately 1 balishta or 9 inches) and soak it in saline water. (There are special threads available for Sutra Neti practice)
- Now, sit in Kagasana and insert this through one of the nostrils so that it comes out of the mouth. Then grab both ends of the thread and gently rub back and forth, this way the entire nasal-mouth canal gets cleaned. This is called Neti by the Siddhas.
- Repeat with the other nostril.
- As per Hatharatnavali (1:38) once the thread has been pulled out of the mouth the two ends should be joined and the thread should be rotated through the nasal passage and mouth.
- Throughout the whole practice keep breathing through the mouth.
- Sutra Neti can be practiced every day if you are suffering from sinusitis, cold, insensitivity to smell, headache, eye strain, or

eye infection. Otherwise, it is best to practice only once a week and then once a month.

GS also mentioned Sutra Neti.

Benefits-

- Neti cleanses the cranium and bestows clairvoyance. It also destroys all diseases which manifest above the throat. The practice of Neti promotes a balance between the left and right nostrils and consequently the right and left-brain hemispheres.
- Neti exerts a relaxing and irrigating effect upon the eyes by stimulating the tear ducts and glands.
- The membrane lining the nostril secrets a protective film of sticky mucus. Tiny hairlike cilia promote the movement of mucus, along with pollutants, dust, etc. The nasal membrane is highly innervated by nerve fibers and is perhaps the most sensitive area of the whole body.
- These nerve fibers include not only the fibers of the olfactory nerve (the first cranial nerve) responsible for the sense of smell but also numerous other autonomic fibers that relay information to the brain about the inflowing breath, not only smells but also environmental temperature, humidity, and allergens in the air are all sensed by the nose as the flowing breath is drawn across this mucous membrane.

Contraindication: Excessive blocked nose, and Internal infection

There are some other ways of practicing Neti as well. These are-

1. Jala Neti (Nasal irrigation with water)

2. Dugdha Neti (Nasal irrigation with milk)

3. Ghrita Neti (Nasal irrigation with clarified butter)

Out of these, Dugdha Neti and Ghrita Neti are only to be practiced under the advice and supervision of a therapist. **Jala Neti might be the most popular way of practicing Neti kriya.**

Process-

Make saline water, and fill the neti pot.

Sit in Kagasana and put the nozzle of the pot in one of the nostrils, tilt the head slightly and start pouring the water in.

The water will start to come out of the other nostril.

Repeat with the other nostrils.

Once the kriya is done, sit in any comfortable asana and do Kapalbhati to ensure that there is no water remaining in the nostrils.

To ensure this, make a fist with the right hand and exhale on the back of the palm. You will see the water droplet coming out of the nostrils.

> Once you see no more water droplets then rub the throat, sinuses, back of the ears, and forehead, a couple of times to ensure all the water is evaporated. This can be practiced every day to begin with and then later on once or twice a week.
>
> During Jala Neti, if you experience pain in the nose during practice, the quantity of salt is incorrect. Too little salt will create pain and too much salt will cause a burning sensation.

Trataka (Concentrated Gazing)
The practice is same in both HYP and GS.

Looking intently with an unwavering gaze at a small point until tears are shed is known as Trataka. There are 2 forms of the practice- **Bahiranga Trataka** - Gazing at an object, **Antaranga Trataka** - Clear and stable inner visualization of an object.

Trataka is done with various objects. The most commonly practiced way is **Jyoti Trataka** or candle gazing because even after closing the eyes, the impressions of the flame remain for some time and Antaranga Trataka can be easily practiced.

Other symbols or objects used are a crystal ball, shiva lingam, yantra, mandala, full moon, a star, the rising or setting sun (orange ball not yellow), a chakra, the symbol of Om, your own shadow. Trataka can also be done on a rose, a tree, a mountain, the sea, and lightning.

Of all the symbols and objects, the most suitable for general use is a candle flame because a symbol, yantra /mandala leaves an impression in the mind and stimulates particular centers. Trataka can be done at any time, but it is more effective when performed on an empty stomach.

Benefits:

- Trataka eradicates all eye diseases, fatigue, and sloth and closes the doorway creating these problems. **It should be kept secret like a golden casket.**
- This practice can induce telepathy, telekinesis, and psychic healing.
- Further results of Ekagrata are strong willpower, improved memory, and concentration ability.
- Physiologically, Trataka relieves eye ailments such as strain, headache, myopia, astigmatism, and even early stages of cataracts.

Contraindication:

- Epileptics should avoid gazing at flickering candles, they can choose a steady object only.
- If you have insomnia, this practice at night will make your mind wide awake and difficult to go to sleep.
- In the case of a tensional headache, this may aggravate pain.

Nauli (Abdominal Massaging)
HYP mentions only one type of Nauli Kriya

- This is a practice of contracting and isolating the rectus abdominis Muscles.
- Lean forward, protrude the abdomen, and rotate (the muscle) from right to left with speed. This is called Nauli by the Siddhas.

GS mentions 3 types. Here It is called Laukiki.

- The root word Nala means the navel string i.e., rectus abdominal muscles. It also means tubular vessels. Laukiki comes from the word Lola which means to roll or agitate.
- It is done 3 ways-
  - **Dakshin Nauli** - Muscle Rotation from left to right
  - **Vama Nauli** - Muscle Rotation from right to left
  - **Madhyama Nauli** - When the middle group of muscles protrudes.
- **Uddiyana Bandha is preparatory for Nauli.**

Benefits:

- Nauli is the foremost of the hatha yoga practices. It kindles the digestive fire, removing indigestion, sluggish digestion, and all disorders of the doshas, and brings about happiness. It is referred to as the Goddess of creation.
- Asana and Pranayama practice definitely generate energy, but Nauli activates the system in a much shorter time and with greater force.
- It balances the endocrine system and helps control the production of sex hormones.

Contraindication:

Suffering from heart disease, Hypertension, Hernia, Gastric or Duodenal Ulcers, Recovering from some internal injury or abdominal surgery, Pregnancy

Kapalbhati (Frontal Brain Cleansing)

As per HYP, this is a practice of forceful exhalation with passive inhalation like the bellows of a blacksmith.

Perform exhalation and inhalation rapidly like the bellows (of a blacksmith). This is called Kapalbhati and it destroys all mucous disorders.

In GS, this is known as **Bhalbhati** and it is of 3 types.

Bhal- Cranium /Forehead, Bhati- Light / Splendour or perception and knowledge.

Vatakrama- Sit in Padmasana or any other dhyana asana. Keep left palm in Dhyan mudra, and right palm in nasikagra or pranava mudra. Keep the back straight, and chin parallel to the ground. Now close the right nostril with the right thumb and inhale rapidly through the left (Ida). Then immediately close the left nostril and exhale through the right (Pingala). Again, immediately inhale through the right and exhale through the left. Just like a rapid anuloma-viloma, without retention. The last stroke ends on exhaling through the left.

Vyutkrama- Draw water through both the nostrils and expel it through the mouth. Repeat the process multiple times.

Sheet Krama- Suck water by the mouth producing a hissing sound, and throw it out through the nostrils. Repeat the process multiple times.

Benefits (Kapalbhati and Vatakrama)

- During normal inhalation, fluid around the brain is compressed and the brain contracts very slightly. With an exhalation, this **cerebrospinal fluid (CSF)** is decompressed and the brain very slightly expands. This is the mechanical influence of the respiratory cycle on the structure of the brain.
- The forced exhalation nature of Kapalbhati increases the massaging effect on the brain by enhancing the decompression effect on every exhalation.
- The average number of breaths is 15/min. This means the brain is compressed/decompressed that many times, but here you are breathing 50-100 times in a min, stimulating the brain 3-7 times more than normal per minute.
- Kapalbhati helps relax facial muscles and nerves. It rejuvenates tired cells and nerves, keeping the face young, shining, and wrinkle-free.
- Kapalbhati is a kriya that invigorates the entire brain and awakens the dormant centers which are responsible for subtle perception. It helps to get rid of Kapha Dosha

Contraindication:

High or low blood pressure, heart disease, Gastric ulcers, Hernia, Epilepsy, Vertigo, Migraine, Significant Nosebleeds, Detached retina, Glaucoma, History of stroke, Recent abdominal surgery, Pregnancy

Hatha Yoga Pradipika is written by Sage Swatmaram Suri. The structure of practices suggested by him is known as **Chaturanga yoga** as it has 4 limbs- **Asana, Pranayama, Mudra & Bandha and Nadanusandhana**
Gheranda Samhita is a collection of teaching by Sage Gheranda to his disciple Chandrakapali. The structure suggested by him is known as **Saptanga Yoga** as it has 7 limbs - **Shatkarma, Asana, Mudra, Pratyahara, Pranayama, Dhyana, and Samādhi.** It is also known as **Ghatasya Yoga.**

1.11 Concept and principles of Yogasana:

Meaning, definition, types and their significance in Yoga Sadhana

Yogasana

Undoubtedly **Yogasana** is the most popular aspect of yoga practice. Asana practice brings **Dridhta (strength)** to the body. A consistent asana practice ensures that the body remains disease-free and the prana flows freely so that the individual can function at its fullest.

Yogasana also prepares the body for higher spiritual practices. One can only sit in dhyana for a longer duration once there is no illness in the body and it is strong enough to stay in one posture.

In Patanjali Yoga Sutra Sage Patanjali mentions a very interesting benefit of doing Asana. He says Asana can help to overcome dualities. Interestingly there are only 3 sutras dedicated to Asana practice in PYS and there is no name of any particular asana.

Sthira Sukham Asanam ||PYS 2.46||
Prayatna-Shaithilya-Ananta-Samapatti-bhyam ||PYS 2.47||
Tato-Dvandva-Anabhighatah ||PYS 2.48||

Refer to Unit 2.4 for the explanation of these sutras,

In Hatha Yoga, asana means something else. Asana is a specific position that opens the energy channels and psychic centers. Hatha Yoga is a process through which purification and control of the body take place by restructuring the flow of prana. The Hatha yogis also found that by developing control of the body through asana, the mind is controlled. Therefore, asana practice is foremost in hatha yoga. When you practice asana, steadiness develops, Prana moves freely, and there is less chance of disease occurrence.

The yogic tradition says that in all, there are 84 lakhs of asanas.

Principles:

- As Patanjali says, Prayatna Shaithilya, means relaxed efforts. The asana should be performed with ease. One should understand that it takes time to master any asana so stay patient.
- Most of the asana focuses on spinal mobility. There are 5 kinds of Spine movements - **Elongation, Twisting, Lateral Bending, Forward Bending, and Arching.** The Asana practice should involve all these movements. Remember the saying in the yoga

community, we are **as young as the spine is flexible**, so keep the spine flexible.

- Always follow the correspondent breathing technique to the asana. For example, in Padahastasana, or Standing Forward Fold, one has to exhale and go in the posture; once you reach the Padahastasana then, you can start to breathe normally. In Bhujangasana, one has to inhale and go into the asana, then one needs to breathe normally.
- The posture should be released exactly the way you went into the posture. **Last in first out.** Remember an asana is not over until it is released comfortably.

Types of Asanas- Asanas are primarily classified as **meditative, Cultural, and Relaxative**

Meditative Asanas- These are sitting postures, which maintain the body in a steady and comfortable condition. Such as, Siddhasana, Swastikasana, Padmasana, Vajrasana, and Sukhasana etc.

Cultural Asanas- These involve static stretching, which brings about the proper tone of muscles. They contribute to the flexibility of the spine and keep the back and spinal muscles stronger. They also stimulate the proper working of the vital organs in the thoracic and abdominal cavities. There are innumerable Cultural Asanas, which are performed through sitting, lying, and standing positions such as - Pavan Muktasana, Naukasana, Vipareeta Karni, Sarvang asana, Matsyasana, Halasana, Chakrasana, Trikonasana, etc.

Relaxative Asanas- These involve relaxing asanas such as Shavasana, Makarasana, Balasana, etc. They are performed in the lying position and are meant for giving rest to the body and mind.

There is another categorization of types of Asanas-

Standing- Such as Tadasana, Vrikshasana, Trikonasana etc.

Sitting- Such as Sukhasana, Paschimottasana, Padmasana, Mandukasana etc.

Prone- Such as Makarasana, Bhujangasana, Shalabhasana, Dhanurasana etc.

Supine- Such as Pawanmuktasana, Ardha Halasana, Chakrasana etc.

Topsy-Turvy- Such as Sarvangasana, Sheersasana, Vrishchikasana

Stages and Phases - Approach phase, Asana phase, Returning phase

Health Benefits:

- Yogasana improves strength, balance, and flexibility.
- Yogasana helps with back pain relief.
- Yogasana can ease arthritis symptoms.
- Yogasana benefits heart health.
- Yogasana helps in easing menstrual pain.
- It is highly recommended for pregnant women.
- Yogasana relaxes you and helps in improving the sleep quality.

> **Tips For Breathing Pattern-**
>
> Remember that whenever your chest is opened up you have to inhale and whenever your chest is contracted then you have to exhale. Such as in postures like Bhujangasana, Hastottanasana, Ardha Chakrasana, etc., the chest gets opened hence we have to inhale while going into the posture. Whereas in postures like Padahastasana, Paschimottanasana, Parvatasana, etc the chest is contracted hence we have to exhale while going into the posture.
>
> Now, whenever you are twisting or bending always use the exhales. For instance, In Katichakrasana Inhale first and then exhale and twist. Same with Bhoo Namanasnaa- Inhale, exhale and then twist. Another example can be Trikonasana, Inhale, and exhaling bend. Try experiencing this by yourself and you will understand the breathing patterns for all the asanas.

1.12 Concept and principles of Pranayama:

Meaning, definition, types and their significance in Yoga Sadhana

Pranayama:

The word Prana is a combination of two syllables, **Pra and Na. Prana denotes constancy**, it is a force that is in constant motion. The literal meaning of the word Pranayama is –

Prana- Vital Force and Ayama - To Stretch or to expand.

Hence the process of expanding the vital force is referred to as Pranayama. It is not merely breath control, but a technique through which the quantity of prana in the body is activated to a higher frequency. Breathing is a direct means of absorbing prana and the manner in which we breathe sets off pranic vibrations which influence our entire being.

Elements of pranayama

Typically, there are 3 elements of pranayama-

- Puraka (Inhalation)
- Rechaka (Exhalation)
- Kumbhaka (Retention)
  - Antara Kumbhaka (Internal Retention)
  - Bahya Kumbhaka (External Retention)
  - Kevala Kumbhaka (A transcendental Kumbhaka, which occurs spontaneously through the regular practice of pranayama).

Types of Breathing

Before we begin the practice of Pranayama, it's important to build awareness of the breath. A normal breath is distinguished by three phases- **Inhalation, exhalation, and pause after exhalation**. When these three are put together, it is known as **respiration.**

Quiet, rhythmic, and deep breathing plays a very important role in our health. It has a harmonizing and calming effect on the body and mind. On the other hand, breathing that is too rapid and shallow has a negative influence on us, as it can intensify nervousness, stress, tension, and pain. Usually, there are **three different channels** through which one breathes. These are-

Through Abdomen / Diaphragmatic Breathing- This is the most natural way of breathing. In this channel Inhalation pushes the diaphragm down, thereby releasing the abdominal organs outwards which results in the expansion of the belly. Exhalation pulls the diaphragm upwards which flattens the abdomen. Abdominal breathing optimizes the capacity of the lungs and makes the breath rhythmic and relaxing. **The infants effortlessly breathe in this way. Even adults while asleep breath this way.**

Through Chest/Thoracic Breathing- In thoracic breathing, there is heaving of the chest or rib cage. The rib cage expands in all directions with inhalation and with exhalation, the ribs revert to their original position. In this type of breathing, the intake of Oxygen is lower than the abdominal breathing and the breath tends to be faster. **Most of us use only this channel for routine breathing.** Apart from that in moments of stress and worry, our breathing becomes heavily chest oriented. The unconscious use of this more rapid form of breathing creates a heightened state of tension. To break this unfavorable cycle, slow and deep abdominal breathing is of great assistance.

Through Collarbone/Clavicular Breathing- In this type of breathing air flows into the top of the lungs. With inhalation, the upper part of the chest and collarbone gets lifted and with exhalation, they come lower. The breath in this breathing is **very shallow and rapid.** Clavicular breathing occurs in situations of extreme stress and panic or when one is having great difficulty in breathing.

All these 3 channels are **significant** and sometimes can be very crucial for our **survival**. In Yoga, there is special emphasis given to strengthening these individual channels. This is referred to as **Sectional Breathing.**

Abdomen/Diaphragmatic Breathing- This breathing is complemented with Dhyana mudra/Chin Mudra.

- Sit in Sukhasana, Padmasana, or Vajrasana and keep the palms in dhyana mudra. Place the palms on the knees. Elbows will be touching the body.
- Inhale filling the stomach with as much air as you can. The stomach should bulge out.
- Then exhale slowly, emptying the stomach completely.
- Repeat 5-10 times.

Thoracic Breathing- This breathing is complemented with Chinmayi mudra.

- Sit in Sukhasana, Padmasana, or Vajrasana and keep the palms in Chinmaya mudra. Palms will be facing upwards and placement would be on the middle of the thighs. Elbows will be touching the body. This placement of the palms ensures that the chest opens up.
- Now, inhale slowly by expanding the chest as much as possible.
- Exhale slowly by contracting the chest.
- The focus is only on the chest expansion and contraction, not on the stomach
- Repeat 5-10 times.

Clavicular Breathing- This breathing is complemented with Adi mudra.

- Sit in Sukhasana, Padmasana, or Vajrasana and keep the palms in Adi mudra. Palms will be facing upwards and placement would be at the crease of the thighs, where the upper and lower body meets. Elbows will be touching the body. This placement of the palms ensures that the shoulders are raised a little.
- Inhale lifting the shoulders up, and Exhale while bringing the shoulder down.
- The focus is only on the shoulder movement and throat breathing, not on the chest or stomach.
- Repeat 5-10 times.

Full Yogic Breath- This breathing is complemented with Bhairavi/ Bhairava mudra.

One full yoga breath includes one smooth, continuous flow of breath in and out, involving non-jerky movements of the abdomen, chest, and collarbone.

Imagine filling the water in a pot. As we pour in the water, the bottom of the pot gets filled at first. While emptying the pot, the bottom of the pot gets emptied last.

We will use the same analogy while performing the Yogic breath.

Process

- Sit in Sukhasana, Padmasana, or Vajrasana and keep the palms in Bhairavi (Females) / Bhairava (Males) mudra. Palms will be facing upwards, and placement will be below the navel. Elbows will be touching the body.

- As you inhale, the stomach bulges out first, then the chest expands, and at last, the throat will be filled which will be complemented by raising the shoulders a little.
- As you exhale, lower the shoulders first, contract the chest, and then empty the stomach.
- These concepts of sectional breathing and full yogic breath should be practiced in building awareness of the breath in a yoga class. One can begin the class with this (after prayer). This should also be done before practicing any pranayama.

Nadi Shodhan Pranayama/Anuloma - Viloma

This is not part of the traditionally suggested Pranayama / Kumbhakas in Hatha yoga texts, instead, **it is mentioned separately**. HYP as well as GS, both texts say that before beginning the pranayama/Kumbhakas, one should clean the Nadis by Nadi Shodhan Pranayama.

In Gherand Samhita, it is mentioned that if Nadis are blocked then the prana or the vital force won't be able to flow properly. Nadi Shodhan Pranayama ensures the proper functioning of the Nadi channel.

It is ideal to perform Nadi Shodhan Pranayama before the pranayama practice. Also, the text says that the practitioner should face either **east or north** while practicing this. In ancient times yogis used to use a mat made of Kusha grass or the skin of deer or lion. But let's not go that far, instead using a blanket or cotton mat is also okay.

Technique:

Nadi Shodhan Pranayama as per HYP

- Sit in Padmasana (This is the most suggested posture as per HYP, but any meditative posture is okay)
- Keep the right hand in either Pranava or Nasikagra mudra. The left hand remains in Dhyan or Chin mudra.
- Close the right nostril with the right thumb, and inhale through the left nostril (Ida), Post inhaling through the Ida, hold the breath to capacity, and then exhale through the right nostril (Pingala).
- Then again inhale through the right nostril, hold the breath up to capacity, and exhale through the left nostril.
- This is one round.
- The basic ratio of Inhale: Retention: Exhale (Puraka: Kumbhaka: Rechaka) is 1:4:2. The idea is to reduce the movement of the breath and to increase the duration of the breath, which is why the retention count is higher.
- The count that we usually practice is 4:16:8. The highest count as per the texts can be 20:80:40.
- Once the practitioner is thorough with this ratio then a Bahya Kumbhaka can be added after exhale, which should be 3 times the inhale. So, the ratio now becomes- Inhale: Internal Retention: Exhale: External Retention- 1:4:2:3. The highest count can be 20:80:40:60.
- Beginners or people with heart diseases/ lung issues should practice Anuloma-Viloma without retention. Then they can slowly build up the strength for retention.

- Swatmaram says that through the regular practice of Nadi Shodhan Pranayama, a Yogi can purify all the Nadis within three months.

Nadi Shodhan Pranayama as per GS

In Gherand Samhita Nadi Shodhan is done in two ways, **Samanu and Nirmanu.**

Samanu- This is done with the Beeja mantra.

- First, inhale through the left nostril while chanting the beeja mantra for **Vayu "Yam"** 16 times then hold your breath in (Antah- Kumbhaka) while chanting the "Yam" 64 times and exhale through the right nostril while chanting "Yam" 32 chants.
- Now inhale through the right nostril while chanting the Beeja mantra for **fire "Ram",** 16 times, then hold your breath while chanting the "Ram" 64 times and exhale through the left nostrils while chanting "Ram" 32 times.
- Then think of the moon on the tip of the nose and inhale again through the left nostril while chanting "**Tham**" 16 times, then hold the breath in for 64 chants of "**Vam**" and exhale through the right while chanting "**Lam**" 32 times.

Nirmanu- Cleaning the Nadis with Dhauti karma is referred to as Nirmanu.

Types of Pranayama / Kumbhaka- Pranayama is referred as Kumbhaka in HYP and GS.

HYP mentions 8 types of Kumbhaka- **Surya Bhedana, Ujjayi, Seetkari, Sheetali, Bhastrika, Bhramri, Moorchha, and Plavini**

GS also mentions 8 types of Kumbhaka-**Sahita (Sagarbha and Nigarbha), Surya Bhedana, Ujjayi, Sheetali, Bhastrika, Bhramri, Moorchha, and Kevali**

Science of effects of breath on the internal body:

The breathing process is directly related to the brain. It is one of the most vital processes in the body. As stated in Hatha Yoga Pradipika-

Chale- Vatam- Chale- Chittam- Nishchale- Nishchalam- Bhavet | Yogi- Sthanutvam- Apnoti - Tato- Vayum- Nirodhyet ||HYP||

Meaning- When prana moves, Chitta (the mental force) moves, when prana is without movement, Chitta is without movement. By this (steadiness of prana) the yogi attains steadiness and should thus restrain the Vayu.

The breathing process has a direct impact on the central nervous system and also has some connections with the hypothalamus, the brain center which controls emotional responses.

The hypothalamus is responsible for transforming perception into cognitive experience. Erratic breathing sends erratic impulses to this center and thus creates disturbed responses.

There are also certain areas of the nasal mucous membrane which are connected to the visceral organs. When impulses coming from the nose are arrhythmic, the visceral organs, particularly those connected to the coccygeal plexus, respond in the same manner, arrhythmically.

Being disturbed, these organs again send irregular impulses to the brain and cause more disharmony and imbalance. This is a continuous cycle. By becoming aware of the nature of the breath and by restraining it, the whole system becomes controlled.

Importance of retention

Pranayama is usually considered to be the practice of controlled inhalation and exhalation combined with retention. Retention is given very much importance because it allows a longer period of assimilation of prana, just as it allows more time for the exchange of oxygen and carbon-di-oxide in the cells

When you retain the breath, you are stopping nervous impulses in different parts of the body and harmonizing the brain wave patterns. The longer the breath is held, the greater the gap between nerve impulses and their responses to the brain. When retention is held for a prolonged period, mental agitation decreases.

Health Benefits of Pranayama

- Through Pranayama one would be able to reduce the breathing rate. A reduced breathing rate has the direct effect of slowing down the heart rate, improving blood circulation, lowering blood pressure, and slowing down the aging process.
- Pranayama improves lung diffusion capacity. Pranayama is highly suggested for respiratory disorders such as Asthma, allergic rhinitis, Covid, etc.
- Yogic breathing practices increase the levels of leptin, a hormone produced by fat tissues that signal the brain to inhibit hunger.
- Pranayama practice may help overcome insomnia, migraine, or any disorders which occur due to the absence of proper

relaxation. This can also be very helpful for people who are trying to quit an addiction such as cigarettes, alcohol, food, etc.
- Pranayama practice requires being aware of the breath which results in being more mindful.

Concept of Panch Prana

There are 5 main Vayu functions as per Prashnopanishad- **Apana, Prana, Samana, Udana, and Vyana.**

Samana is considered the highest form of Vayu. Maitri Upanishad says Samana is a higher form of Vyana and between them is the production of Udana.

Sitting postures for pranayama- Siddhasana, Padmasana and Ardha Padmasana, Swastikasana, Sukhasana, and Vajrasana.

1.13 Introduction to Tri Bandha

Jalandhar bandha (Throat Lock)

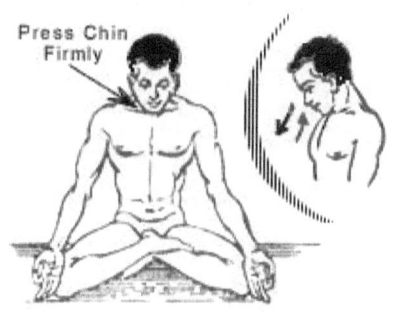

Contracting the throat by bringing the chin to the chest in Antar Kumbhaka / Bahya Kumbhaka, is called Jalandhar Bandha. This stimulates Vishuddhi Chakra. There are **2 interpretations** of its name

- Jalan means net and Dhara means stream or flow. The Jalandhara bandha is the lock that controls the network of Nadis in the neck. The physical manifestations of these Nadis are the blood vessels and nerves in the neck.
- Alternatively- Jal means water. Jalandhara bandha is therefore the throat lock that holds the nectar or fluid flowing down to Vishuddhi from Bindu and prevents it from falling into the digestive fire. This is the way to boost the prana reservoir.

Practice

- Sit in any Siddhasana, Sidhayoni asana, Padmasana, Vajrasana or Sukhasana. Place the palm on the knees.
- Inhale and retain the breath and lower the chin against the chest in a way that you start feeling the pressure on the throat.

- Simultaneously, straighten and lock the elbows, press the knees down with the hands, and hunch the shoulders upwards and forward. Hold your breath for as long as you can.
- Then slowly bring the chin parallel to the ground, relax the shoulders, and exhale slowly through the nostrils

Benefits

- The practice of this Bandha destroys all throat-related disorders. Removes old age and gives victory over death.
- Improves the functioning of the thyroid and parathyroid glands.
- Regular practice induces mental relaxation and relieves anxiety, stress, and hunger.

Contraindications- Cervical spondylosis, High intracranial pressure, Vertigo, Heart disease

Uddiyana Bandha

The word "Uddiyana" means **"to rise up" or "to fly upward"**. This practice causes the diaphragm to rise towards the chest, hence the name. Uddiyana is often translated as the stomach lift. Another meaning is that the physical lock helps to direct prana into Sushumna Nadi so that it flows upward to the Sahasra chakra. Uddiyana Bandha is practiced in Bahya Kumbhaka only. It stimulates the Manipura chakra.

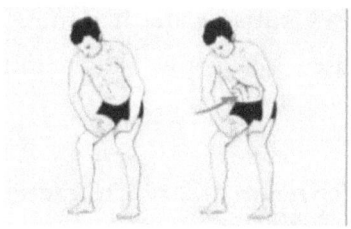

Preparation- Uddiyana bandha must be practiced on an empty stomach. The bowels should be empty. Agnisara Kriya is an excellent preparatory practice.

Practice

- Stand tall with feet shoulder-width distance apart. Inhale through the nostrils and exhale bending forward from the waist, bringing the upper body parallel to the ground.
- Hold your breath out. Place the palms on the knees and keep the arms straight.
- Keeping the breath out, contract the abdomen muscles upwards and inwards towards the spine. Hold the lock for as long as possible, without straining.
- Slowly raise the body up, exhale slightly to release the lock on the lungs, and then slowly inhale through the nose.
- The same can be practiced sitting as well.

Benefits-

- The practice of this bandha destroys old age and helps one to conquer death.
- Stimulates digestive fire. Stimulates all the abdominal organs.
- Stimulates the solar plexus.

Contraindications- Colitis, Stomach or Intestinal ulcers, Hernia, HBP, Heart disease, Glaucoma, High intracranial pressure, Pregnancy.

Moola Bandha (Perineum / Cervix retraction lock)

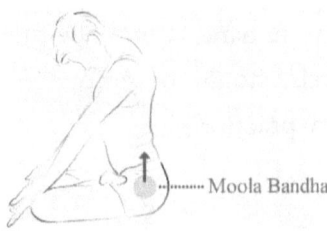
Moola Bandha

The word Moola means root / firmly fixed. Mooladhar refers to the root of the spine or the perineum where the seat of the kundalini or the primal energy is locked. Moola Bandha is effective in activating Mooladhar Chakra.

It is important to understand that moola bandha is a contraction of **specific muscles in the pelvic floor**, not the entire pelvic floor.

In the male body, the area of contraction **is between the anus and the testes.**

In the female body, the area of contraction is **behind the cervix**, where the uterus projects into the vagina.

With practice one becomes aware of these regions. **Ashwini and Vajroli** mudras can be performed as preparation for the Mooladhar bandha.

Practice

- Sit in a comfortable meditative asana, preferably Siddha / Siddha yoni asana.
- Close your eyes and bring awareness to the perineal. Inhale and hold your breath in, and contract the perineal/vaginal region by pulling up the muscles of the pelvic floor. Hold for as long as possible.
- Slowly release the bandha and exhale.
- Moola Bandha is usually practiced with Jalandhara Bandha in Antah kumbhak.
- Beginners can also practice rhythmic contraction and relaxation of pelvic floor muscles with normal breathing to build awareness and strength.

Benefits-

- Stimulates the pelvic nerves and tones the urogenital and excretory system.
- Induces sexual control.
- Destroys old age.
- Makes one grounded and stable.

Contraindication- Menstruation, Piles, HBP.

Maha Bandha (The Great Lock)

All the above-mentioned bandhas, when employed together is called Maha Bandha

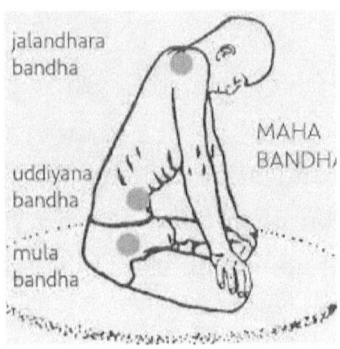

Practice

- Place the left heel firmly at the region between the anus and penis (Perineum). Having placed the right foot on the left thigh.
- Then after inhalation performs Jalandhar bandha, moola bandha, and turn the mind into Shambhavi mudra. The air should be exhaled slowly after doing Kumbhak repeat with another side.
- As per Jyotsna (Commentary on HYP)- The Moolbandha happens by itself on the application of jiva bandha hence there is no need to apply Moolbandha once Jivhabandha is applied.
- Some guru says that there is no need for Jalandhar bandha. Applying Jivhabandha by pressing the tongue at the center of the Rajdanta (tooth) is comparatively simple.
- In Hatha Yoga Pradipika, Maha bandha. is explained in 2 ways-
  - With Antah Kumbhak, applying Jalandhar Bandha, Mool Bandha, and Shambhavi Mudra.
  - With Bahya Kumbhak, applying Jalandhar, Uddiyana, and Moola Bandha.

Benefits

- Mahabandha is the bestower of great siddhis.
- This frees one from bonds of death and makes the 3 nadis unite in Ajna chakra.
  - **As per HYP Mahabandha should be performed with Mahamudra and Mahavedha mudras for the utmost benefits**

Contraindication – Same as each bandha.

1.14 Dhyana and its significance in health and well-being

Dhyana means Meditation. According to Patanjali, **"Uninterrupted flow (of mind) towards the chosen object (for meditation) is Dhyana."** Dhyana is a transcendental state that happens through the continuous practice of Pratyahara (Withdrawal of senses) and Dharna (Concentration towards one object). With regular practice, one would transcend from "Trying to concentrate" to a "Fully concentrated on the object" state.

One common myth about Dhyana is that it is a practice to make the mind thoughtless whereas it is the practice of directing the thoughts toward the chosen object. Dhyana enables the practitioner to have voluntary control over the thoughts.

There are various forms of Meditation Techniques to suit different levels of practitioners. Such as, Breath observation, Auto-suggestion, Visualization, Mantra chanting, Rotation of beads in Japa, Concentration on an object of choice, and Non-judgmental awareness of thought.

Common meditation techniques-

1. Concentration Mediation

- In this technique, one needs to choose an object as a point of concentration such as breath, the deity (Ishta devata), a candle flame, a mantra, etc. The entire attention is then focused on that object.
- At first, there will be sense distractions (distraction due to the 5 senses) but as one would continue practicing, the Pratyahara (voluntary withdrawal of senses) would happen.

- Then the state of Dharna would be conquered by fully occupying the mind with the thoughts of the objects only.
- Then one would transcend to a state of uninterrupted flow towards the object, i.e., Dhyana.

> Dhyana practices should not be suggested to people who are clinically depressed. The overthinking pattern of such practitioners might increase when they are pushed to close their eyes and asked to focus on something. The flow of destructive thoughts will be unconsciously higher in such practitioners. The ideal yogic approach for people who are in a state of depression/excessive overthinking is to teach them physical practices such as Surya Namaskara, Hrid Gati, Sarvanga Pushti, etc. Special attention should be given to increasing mobility of the upper back, shoulders, and neck because the pain in these areas is one of the prime physical manifestations of stress. As the practitioner starts to feel better with their physical health, they can be taught Sectional breathing, and full yogic breath.

2. Mindfulness Meditation

- In practicing mindful meditation, one is needed to let the thoughts come and go into the mind, but remain fully unaffected by them.
- One needs to watch the flow of their own thoughts as a third person. They need to watch the evolution and dissolution of their thoughts on their own.

- This is a very important practice that teaches you the power a thought can have over oneself and how powerless the thought becomes when one stops identifying with it.
- All the emotions that one feels are merely the effect of thoughts. The moment the thought is taken over by another thought the emotion also vanishes. For instance, if a spouse is angry with another that anger quickly goes away when their infant chuckles or does any funny movement.
- To gain voluntary control over thoughts, Patanjali suggests a practice called **Pratipaksha Bhavana,** which advocates keeping the opposite thoughts when any destructive or negative thought comes into the mind. Such as when we feel anger towards someone comes, voluntarily bring a thought of love.

Health benefits of Dhyana

- It makes you aware of yourself, increases intuition, keeps you calm, and enhances compassion, empathy, and kindness. Works as a natural stress stabilizer.
- It develops the willpower needed to avoid bad habits.
- Meditation practice improves the brain's problem-solving and decision-making strategies.
- Research shows that meditators have lower cortisol levels in the brain which explains their insightful nature and resilience.
- A study on the effect of an 8-week mindful meditation course found that people who are regular meditation practitioners had heightened attention and concentration span.

1.15 Introduction to Yogic relaxation techniques with special reference to Yoga Nidra

Yoga Nidra- Yogic sleep is a state of consciousness between waking and sleeping, like the "going-to-sleep" stage, The practice is typically induced by guided meditation. This is a progressive movement of self-awareness and promotes a sense of physical, emotional, and mental relaxation. The practice of Yoga Nidra at the end of the session makes one feel rejuvenated even after an advanced class.

The practice is largely taught and promoted by **Swami Satyanand Saraswati of the Bihar School of Yoga.** There are various techniques but general instructions will be like these-

Prep

- Lie down in savasana with your feet open shoulder width apart and palms facing the ceiling, eyes closed.
- Do not resist any pull of gravity, surrender.

Practice

- Now with a very aware state of mind, move your attention to your right foot, right calf, right thigh, right hip, right side of the stomach, right chest, right side of the back, right shoulder, right upper arm, right forearm, right palm, right fingers, right thumb, Be aware.
- Now pay attention to your left foot, left calf, left thigh, left hip, the left side of the stomach, left chest, the left side of the back, left shoulder, left upper arm, left forearm, left palm, left fingers, and left thumb.

- Pay attention to the neck, sides of the neck, back of the neck, and throat.
- Pay attention to the face, chin, cheeks, nose, ears, eyes, and forehead.
- Pay attention to the crown.
- Pay attention to the entire body from head to toe, and repeat in your mind- I am healthy, I am strong, I am calm, I am having a nice day today.
- Stay with yourself focusing on the breath. (Pause for 30 sec)

Returning Phase

- Now bring your awareness back to the surroundings. Be aware of the place you are in and the people around you.
- Make movements of your toes and, fingers.
- Move your neck from side to side.
- Turn your body to one side, take the support of the floor, and sit up on the mat. Keep the eyes still closed.

From here you can either do pranayama or end the class with mantra chanting too.

There are 3 more popular relaxation techniques- IRT, QRT, and DRT.

IRT- (Instant Relaxation Technique)-

This is the practice of **progressive contraction and relaxation** of several muscles in the body. This is usually done at the beginning of the Yoga class and usually takes 2-3 minutes however, it can also be done any time of the day to induce relaxation. The practice helps in strengthing mind-body awareness along with releasing any tension built in the muscles.

The ideal posture for IRT is Shavasana however it can also be done in a comfortable seated posture.

General Instruction:

- Lie Down in Shavasana
- Take a few slow, deep breaths to center yourself and prepare for the practice. Inhale deeply through your nose, and exhale slowly through your mouth.
- Focus on your toes, curling them downward to tense the muscles in your feet and calves. Hold briefly, then release and let them relax completely. Feel the tension draining away.
- Progressively tense and release each muscle group as you work your way up the body, including the calves, thighs, and buttocks. Hold each tension for a few seconds before releasing.
- Continue by tensing and relaxing the muscles in your abdomen, chest, shoulders, arms, and hands. Pay attention to the sensations of tension and relaxation with each movement. While contracting the abdomen breath would be in **Bahya kumbhaka (External Retention).**
- Lastly, tense the muscles in your neck by gently pressing your head back into the surface you're lying on. Then, scrunch your facial muscles tightly for a few seconds before releasing.
- Take a moment to scan your entire body, from head to toe, noticing any remaining areas of tension. If you find any, gently tense and release those muscles once more to encourage further relaxation.
- Chant Om 2-3 times and observe the vibrations across the body.
- This is one round. One can do 2-3 rounds of this practice.

QRT – (Quick Relaxation Technique)-

This is the practice of **consciousness observation of the breath**. In a yoga class, this practice is usually done after standing postures and takes 5-6 minutes. The practice is very effective in building breath awareness.

General Instruction:

- Lie down in Shavasana. Close your eyes if it feels comfortable.
- Take a moment to settle into the posture, allowing your body to fully release tension and sink into the floor. Feel supported by the earth beneath you.
- Begin by observing the breath as you continue breathing in and out through the nostrils. Observe the natural rise and fall of the abdomen with every breath.
- As you continue to watch the natural movements of your abdomen, gradually deepen the breath by consciously expanding the belly on the inhale and contracting it on the exhale. Allow the breath to flow smoothly and effortlessly.
- Maintain awareness of the breath and the movement of the abdomen. Notice the sensations of expansion and contraction with each breath cycle, staying present in the moment.
- Imagine all the toxins, negativity, tension, etc getting expelled from the body with every exhale, and positivity, prana, and life entering in the body with every inhale.
- As the breath becomes more centered and slow, a natural relaxation with a natural smile will follow
- Continue for 8-10 Rounds.
- Complement every round with chanting Om.

DRT – (Deep Relaxation Technique)-

This technique involves **"A-kara", "U-kara", and "M-kara"** chanting while focusing on different parts of the body. This practice induces deep relaxation and is usually done at the end of the Yoga Class. It typically takes 15-20 minutes.

General Instruction:

- Lie down in Shavasana.
- Begin by taking a few deep breaths to relax your body and calm your mind.
- Direct your attention to your lower body, including your feet, calves, knees, thighs, hips, and pelvis. Mentally scan this area and consciously release any tension or tightness you may feel.
- Begin chanting the syllable **"A"** while focusing your awareness on lower body. Observe the vibrations of chant in the lower body. Chant 2-3 times.
- Shift your focus to your middle body, including your chest, stomach, back, and arms. Relax these muscles and allow any remaining tension to dissolve.
- Chant the syllable **"U"** while directing your attention to the middle body. Feel the vibrations of the sound resonating within your middle body as you continue chanting. Chant 2-3 times
- Finally, bring your awareness to your face, including your forehead, eyes, nose, cheeks, and mouth. Relax the muscles of your face and let go of any tension you may be holding.

- With your face relaxed, chant the syllable **"M"** while focusing on the vibrations in this area. Maintain the silence after the chant and observe the residual vibrations of the **M** chant.
- After completing the chanting of all three syllables individually, transition to chanting "Om" a couple of times. Allow the sound of "Om" to resonate throughout your entire body, and observe any sensations that arise. Notice the vibrations and the subtle shifts in your state of consciousness.
- When you're ready to conclude the practice, gently return your awareness to your breath. Take a few more deep breaths, gradually reawaken your body and mind. Open your eyes slowly and take a moment to reflect on your experience.

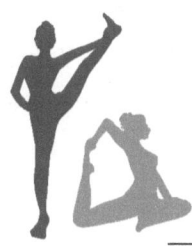

UNIT 2

INTRODUCTION TO YOGA TEXT

2.1 Introduction to Prasthantrayi, Purushartha Chatushtaya, and goal of human life

Prasthantrayi

Vedanta philosophy acknowledges the Prasthantrayi as its **three authoritative sources**. The study of Vedanta is considered incomplete without a close examination of the Prasthantrayi. It collectively refers to-

The Upanishad- These are also referred to as **Sruti Prasthana**. Sruti means that which is heard. It is understood that when rishis sat in deep meditation, they heard the knowledge of the Upanishads.

Bhagavad-Gita- The Bhagavad-Gita is referred to as **Smriti Prasthāna**. Smriti means that which is remembered. This was composed by the sages based on their understanding of the Vedas

Brahma Sutra- The Brahma Sutra is referred to as **Nyaya /Yukti Prasthana.** This is the logical text that sets forth the philosophy systematically.

Purushartha Chatushtaya

Before we study Purushartha Chatushtaya, let's look at the division of human life as per the Indian philosophical viewpoint. Human life is understood to be of 100 years. These 100 years are divided into **4 phases/ashramas -**

Brahmacharya/Student life - 25 years, **Grihastha / Householder** - 25-50 years, **Vanaprastha/Forest dweller** - 50-75 years, and **Sanyasi/Renunciate** - 75-100 Years

Purusha means person or self and Artha means the aim or goal of human life.

The concept of **Purushartha** basically indicates different values to be realized at different stages/ashramas of human life through human efforts. Human life without purpose would be meaningless. One needs to have an end or purpose in life towards which our actions can be directed.

There are four Purushartha or goals of life as per Indian philosophy-

Dharma (virtue)- Dharma here means duty. This is the Indian expression of right activities.
- In Mahabharata, it is mentioned as an ethical concept and defined as that which is right and good.
- **In all stages of a man's life either as a student or as a householder, as a forest dweller or an ascetic, dharma has to be accepted as paramount.**

- Dharma is the most important urge and should be developed to regulate both Artha and Kama.

Artha (wealth)- Artha is the attainment of riches and worldly prosperity, profit, and wealth.

- Artha is a powerful urge in human nature.
- Acquisition of means for material well-being is considered a legitimate social and moral purpose. However, if the urge to seek money or possessions is not restricted then it will lead to self- indulgence or greed and will obstruct the way to the highest good i.e., moksha.
- It is given in one of the pali texts, that **"one who enjoys his wealth and does meritorious deeds with it, experiences pleasure and happiness".**
- Kautilya also says **"Wealth and wealth alone is important. Because charity and desire depend on wealth for their realization."**
- Bhagwad Gita gives guidelines for charity saying **"From the wealth you have earned by rightful means, take out one-tenth, and as a matter of duty, give it away in charity. Dedicate your charity for the pleasure of God"**.

Kama (pleasure)- Kama is ordinarily termed as pleasure. Pleasure is defined as "The enjoyment of the appropriate objects by the five senses of hearing, feeling, seeing, tasting and smelling, assisted by the mind together with the soul."

- It is said, that all that man does is inspired by Kama. As Manu regarded Kama as desire, one can say, it is a desire for pleasure.
- It can be a sensuous pleasure, mental pleasure, pleasure from satisfaction of the work, urges for sexual pleasure, etc.

- But once the pleasures are attained then the question comes, **What next?** If one's life is completely purposed towards attaining pleasures then one will get trapped in a never-ending cycle of greed. It's a very dangerous situation, and that is why following Dharma is considered paramount, irrespective of the purpose or stage of life;

Moksha (liberation)- In Bhagavad-Gita, Moksha is mentioned as supreme tranquillity and the highest bliss. It is a delight in the self, contentment with the self, self-satisfaction, and self-fulfillment.

- This is considered the common aim of human life. It is suggested that one should aim to earn and wisely use wealth as well as satisfy desires by sticking to his / her Dharma. Once the material urges are regulated and disciplined one will get self-fulfillment and then start the search for the **supreme bliss / Moksha.**

2.2 Yoga in Kathopnishad, Prashnopanishad, and Tattiryopanishad with special emphasis on Panchakosha Vivek and Ananda Mimamsa.

Yoga in Kathopnishad-

Kathopnishad / Katha Upanishad is part of **Krishna Yajurveda**. It consists of two chapters (Adhyāyas), each divided into three sections (Vallis). This Upanishad has one of the earliest mentions of Yoga.

The story of Nachiketa-

The Upanishad opens with the story of **Vajashrava, also called Aruni Uddalaki Gautama** who was giving away all of his worldly possessions. However, his son Nachiketa sees the charitable sacrifice as a farce, because all those things have already been used to exhaustion, and are of no value to the recipients. Such as the cows which were given away were so old that they couldn't give any milk and could have died anytime. Nachiketa doesn't like this event and asked his father

"Dear father, to whom will you give me away?" He said it a second, and then a third time. His father gets annoyed and angrily said "To Death, I give you away."

As the Upanishad says that Nachiketa does not die but accepts his father's wish, by visiting the abode of **Yama - the deity of death.** Since Yama was not home, Nachiketa waits outside his palace and as a guest go hungry for three nights. When Yama arrives, he sees him waiting and as an apology for this dishonour to the guest he offers 3 wishes to Nachiketa.

- **Nachiketa's first wish** is that Yama discharges him from the abode of death, and sends him back to his family and that his father becomes calm, well-disposed, not resentful, and the same as he was before when he returns. Yama grants the first wish immediately,
- **For his second wish**, Nachiketa asks for the correct way of performing rituals so that human beings can achieve heaven. Yama grants the second wish also immediately.
- **Nachiketa then asks for his third wish**, asking Yama about the doubt that human beings have about "what happens after a person dies? Initially, Yama tries to persuade Nachiketa in asking anything else as the third wish as he says that answer to this question is not easily available to even gods. But Nachiketa

became persistent about this and Yama had to answer the question, which is detailed in the Upanishad.

- Katha Upanishad asserts <u>Atman</u> / Self exists, though it is invisible and full of mystery. It is ancient, and recognizable by <u>Yoga</u> (meditation on one's self). Yoga is a path to the highest goal of man, which is a life of spiritual freedom and liberation.
- In the 6th Valli of the 2nd Adhyaya, the yogic path to Self-knowledge is explained.

Yada Panchavatishthante Jnanani Mansa Sah ||

Buddhischa Na Vicheshtate Tamahuh Parmam Gatim ||2.6.10||

yadā - when, **pañca jñānāni** - the five senses, **manasā Saha** - with the mind, **avtiṣṭhante** - cease and are at rest, **budhiḥ ca** - the Thought, **na vicestati** - ceases from its workings, **tām** - that, **paramām gatim** - the highest state, **āhuḥ** - say thinkers.

<u>Meaning</u> - Only when the mind with thoughts and the five senses stand still, and when Buddhi does not waver, that they call the highest state.

Tam Yoga Miti Manyante Sthiram-indriyam-dharanam ||

Apramttstada-Bhavati-Yogi-Hi-Prabhava-Apyayau||2.6.11||

Sthirām - the state unperturbed, **indriyadhāraṇām** - when the senses are imprisoned in the mind, **tām yogam** - "it is Yoga", **iti manyate** - this they say, **tadā** - then, **apramataḥ bhavati** - (man) becomes very vigilant, **hi** - for, **yogaḥ** - Yoga is, **Prabhavāpyayau** - the birth of things and their ending.

Meaning- The stillness of the senses, and concentration of the mind, is called Yoga, it is not thoughtless and heedless sluggishness, Yoga is creation as well as dissolution

Yoga in Prashnopanishad-

The **Prashnopanishad** is part of the **Atharva Veda.** The Upanishad consists of 6 questions (Prashna), which were asked to **Rishi Pippalada** by **6 disciples** named- **Kabandhin Katyayana, Bhargava Vaidarbhi, Kausalya Asvalayana, Sauryayanin Gargya, Saibya Satyakama, Sukesan Bharadvaja.**

The Upanishad consists of 6 chapters. Each chapter discussed one question-

Prashnopanishad discusses some of the fundamental concepts of Yogic science-

Concept of Pancha Prana- Answering the question asked by **Kausalya Asvalayana, Rishi Pippalada says that -**

- Prana is born of the Atman. As is the shadow in the man so is this Prana in the Atman.
- As a king command his officers, saying to them, Reside in and govern these or those villages, so does this Prana dispose of the other Pranas each for their separate work.
- **Apana** dwells in the anus and the generative organs. It does excretion.
- **Prana** does the sensory life function. It dwells in the eye, the ears, etc.
- **Samana** dwells in the navel. It does the digestive function.
- **Vyana** does the circulation of blood. It is all-pervading.

- **Udana** helps to swallow food and drink. It takes the Jiva to Brahman during deep sleep. It takes the Jiva out of the body during death and conducts him to the other world. It abides in the throat.
- The sun verily is the external Prana. He rises favoring Prana in the eyes. The goddess of the earth attracts (controls) the Apana downwards. The Akasa (ether) between the sun and the earth is Samana. The wind is Vyana. And the fire is Udana.
- A balance between these five pranas is health, and an imbalance results in disease.

Concept of Nadis-

- Atman is in the heart. There are 101 nerve currents (Nadis). Each of these has a hundred branches; again, each of these has 72000 sub-branches. In these, the Vyana moves.
- Again, through one nerve, the Udana, ascending, leads us upwards to the virtuous worlds by good work, to the sinful world by sin, and to the world of men by virtue and sin combined.

Concept of Aum- Answering the 5th question asked by **Saibya Satyakama** Rishi Pippalada

- Om being the - comprehensive sound symbol of Brahman, represents the manifested state of Brahman (the physical world) by its audible sound and the unmanifested state or the absolute Brahman by its inaudible form (the silence which follows the chant).
- Meditating upon the 'A' syllable enlightens the practitioners. After death, The practitioner comes back to the world of men and achieves greatness with austerity, continence, and faith.

- Meditating upon the 2 syllables "**A+U**" leads the practitioner towards the unit of mind. Unity of mind refers to being in the **Sukshma Sharira (The mental body)**. The practitioner is in Sukshma Sharira (after death) and is taken to the **world of the moon** in the sky. After enjoying the grandeur of it, the practitioner comes back into the world of men again.
- Meditating upon the 3 syllables "**A+U+M**" leads the practitioner towards the path of **Karma Mukti**. The practitioner then gets freed from all of the sins. The practitioner is then taken to the **world of Brahma**. From that macrocosmic self, the practitioner beholds the supreme Purusha residing in the heart.

Yoga in Tattiryopanishad-

The **Tattirya Upanishad** is part of the **Krishna Yajurveda**. There is a legend of how this Upanishad came into being. It is said that the great sage Yajnavalkya quarreled with his Guru Vaisampayana. His guru then asked him to return all the Vedic knowledge that he had studied under him. Yajnavalkya vomited the Yajurveda he had learned. The other pupils of Vaisampayana assumed the forms of Tittiris (birds) and swallowed the Veda thus being thrown out or vomited. Therefore, it came to be known as **Tattirya-Samhita.**

This Upanishad is divided into sections called Vallis-

- **Siksha-Valli (Section on instruction)** - In this section, he gives clear instructions to the aspirants on character building. He imparts the rules of right conduct or right living in order to prepare themselves for the attainment of **Brahma-Jnana** or the knowledge of the Self.

- **Brahmananda-Valli (Section on Brahma-bliss)** - This section deals with the bliss of Brahman. The order of creation is described in this Valli.
- **Bhrigu-Valli (Section on Bhrigu)** - This section deals with the story of Bhrigu, son of Varuna, who, under instructions from his father, understood Bliss or Brahman, after undergoing the required penance.

In Tattirya Upanishad, the very popular Panch kosha theory is discussed.

Pancha-kosha Viveka - This concept talks about 5 different sheaths / koshas of human existence. It can be understood as a yogic attempt to understand how the human body functions.

Annamaya Kosha- (The Physical Sheath)-

- The first sheath of human existence is primarily made up of food. All beings are produced from food, whosoever dwells on the earth. All beings live by the food and in the end, they become the food. It can be said that "Food alone is the eldest living being". Therefore, it is called **universal medicine.** Those who worship Brahman as food, they obtain all food.
- Annamaya Kosha consists of five elements (Pancha Bhutas), namely earth (Prithvi), water (Jala or Apa), fire (Agni or Tejas), wind (Vayu), and space (Akash). It is nourished by the gross food that we consume.
- It includes our bones and also the tissues which make up our muscles and organs. It is the lowest vibration of ourselves.

- It is the structure that contains both the prana and the consciousness. If one gets 'stuck' into this layer, then one becomes over-obsessive about form.
- **Asanas, Kshatriyas, and our diet** help in developing and strengthening Annamaya-kosha.

Pranamaya Kosha- (The Breath Sheath)- Inside Annamaya Kosha, there is another sheath called Pranamaya kosha.

- Prana means energy. This kosha is the vital life force that moves through the body. It literally consists of the breath and the five pranas, namely: Prana, Apana, Udana, Samana, and Vyana.
- These forms of prana control various functions within the physical body, and without prana, the body would be lifeless, and unable to move or think. A uniform harmonious flow of Prana to each cell of the Annamaya kosha keeps them alive and healthy.
- Prana is intimately related to the third Kosha- the Manomayakosha which is the Mind and Body. It helps to control our minds. When the Nadis get blocked due to our faulty lifestyle, when the breath is shallow and its flow is not smooth then prana gets disturbed and it causes the mind to become agitated.
- On the other hand, when pranic energy flows slowly and smoothly then the mind becomes calm and peaceful.
- **The practice of pranayama** works directly on this layer. Pranayama is not just a breathing exercise; it helps the prana reach every cell of the body.
- Manomaya Kosha- (The Mental / Psychological Sheath)- Inside Pranamaya-Kosha, there is another sheath called Manomaya

kosha. The **Pranamaya Kosha is the connection between the Annamaya kosha and the Manomaya Kosha.**

- The Mental sheath pertains to the mind and its thought process. These are the actions and reactions of the physical body which are maintained and fed by thoughts, feelings, and emotions. It works through our five senses and leads to our likes and dislikes.
- **Mindfulness** probably is the most effective way of influencing the Manomaya kosha. Apart from the practice of **Yama and Niyama, Pranayama, and Dhyana** practices can be very helpful in strengthening **Manomaya Kosha.**

Vijnanamaya Kosha (The Intellectual Sheath)-

This is inside Manomaya Kosha. Vijnana means **wisdom or subtle knowledge**. It is a higher intelligence that contains knowledge, the power of discernment, intuition, conscience, and will.

- In order to understand the difference between the Manomaya Kosha and Vijnanamaya Kosha, let's look at this example- when the Manomaya Kosha said, ' It is a beautiful rose, I want to have it,' one started instructing the hands to pick up the flower. But then the inner mind said, 'Sorry, I cannot pluck this flower; it does not belong to me; it is from the neighbor's garden,' and you stopped the action. This inner voice that continuously guides us to do or not to do something is the **Vijnanamaya kosha.**
- Hunger, sleep, fear, and procreative instinct are common to man and animals. It is the Buddhi (discriminating faculty) that is special for man. A person who does not have Buddhi is equal to an animal.

- The practice of Dharana, Dhyana, and Jnana yoga, the study of scriptures (Swadhaya), and Ishvara Pranidhana help strengthen Vijnanamaya Kosha.

Anandmaya Kosha (The Bliss Sheath)-

This is final layer, which is inside the Vijnanamaya Kosha. Ananda is a Sanskrit word that means Joy, Bliss. This is the most subtle layer beyond any explanation. It is the core of our being. It is Spiritual.

- Once this kosha is awakened, we feel Blissful. We experience pure delight, ecstasy, and joy. We forget the existence of our gross body as well as our mind. We are transported to the highest level of our being. We become one with the divine, and we experience nothing but Happiness and bliss.
- The step-by-step practice of Ashtanga Yoga, Bhakti Yoga, and Karma Yoga helps in getting in touch with this sheath.

Ananda Mimamsa-

Mimamsa means to inquire. **Anand Mimamsa** is an inquiry into bliss. This can be understood as a study to understand What is happiness? And more importantly, how can we be truly happy? This is discussed in the **Brahmananda Valli** of **Tattiryopanishad**.

What exactly is studied about happiness? The answer is: whether happiness is born of sense contacts between subject and object (as is usually understood) or whether happiness is the very nature of the Self. The Upanishad starts by looking at the sense of enjoyment as the source of happiness.

- There is a **bhokta, an enjoyer** in every experience. The senses and various faculties of the mind are the **enjoyers** of varied experiences in life. While senses experience objects, the mind experiences **feeling or Bhavana**. Mind, ego, and intellect are the three faculties that enjoy experiences like feeling, ownership, and knowledge respectively.
- A simple experience of pleasure could be taken as an example for this purpose. A person eats something and gains some pleasure. His body did the physical act of eating and pleasure is experienced by the tongue. If observed more keenly, the tongue is engaged by the mind to gain that pleasure. When the mind is withdrawn, the experience of pleasure is hardly there – irrespective of how tasty the food is. The body, senses, and mind are engaged in the act at different levels, the ultimate enjoyer being the mind. Here there is something being enjoyed (Bhoga) and an enjoyer (the bhokta) is present too. The state of experience is a manifestation of happiness. There is a glimpse of happiness, but that happiness is in the experience.
- Upanishad gives an example of a young man, physically strong, and bursting with vitality and energy. He is highly educated and morally upright. He doesn't have any causes of misery or unhappiness such as old age, physical weakness, ignorance, or moral corruption. Poverty, of course, is one of the greatest barriers to the fulfillment of desires and so the Upanishad endows this with plenty of cash, all the wealth of the world, in fact. Now imagine the happiness of this person, young, vital, energetic, noble, very highly educated, and extremely wealthy. This is the **unit of human happiness: 'Ekah manusha Ananda'**

- The next question then comes **Is it possible to get even greater happiness?** The Upanishad then compares the human unit of happiness with other worlds like **Manushya Gandharva, Deva Gandharva**, etc. In Manushya-Gandharva-Loka, happiness is one hundred times the maximum happiness possible in a human body.
- The Upanishad speaks of different layers of existence in terms of an ascending ladder of Lokas, or worlds. As one ascends to these higher heavens, happiness is multiplied by a hundred times at each level. In the highest heavens, happiness is millions and billions of times greater than the maximum of human happiness.
- Now, the interesting part is that every time The Upanishad compares the happiness in these worlds, it always asserts that such happiness is also felt by **the follower of Vedas who is untouched by desires.** Even the happiness that is felt in the Supreme Loka (The highest layer of existence, also referred to as Brahma Loka) which is millions and billions of times greater than the maximum human happiness is the same that is felt by a follower of Veda who is untouched by the desires.
- Man, in his ignorance, feels that happiness is due to the enjoyment of a variety of sense objects and spends all his life trying to get happiness out of sense enjoyment.
- Whereas this Upanishad gives the solution for ultimate bliss as the renunciation of desires and following the Veda.
- One who has the deepest conviction of the Vedantic truth, that one's own Self is of the very nature of bliss, and does not hanker after sense pleasures, will get a hundred times the maximum human happiness in this very life, right now! He doesn't have to earn merit and wait for death to go to the

higher heavens. Whatever happiness the worldly man gets out of sensual enjoyments here and hereafter, the all-renouncing sage of the Upanishad gets here and now, **by the very virtue of his renunciation.**

2.3 Study Of Bhagwad Gita

Concept of Sthitaprajna, Bhakti, Karma, and Dhyana in Bhagwad Gita, Significance of Bhagwad Gita in day to day life, Concept of Healthy Living in Bhagwad Gita

Concept of Sthitaprajna-

Sthita - Steady and Prajna- Wisdom. The concept of steady wisdom is discussed extensively in Chapter 2 of the Bhagavad Gita.

arjuna uvācha

sthita-prajñasya kā bhāṣhā samādhi-sthasya Keshava

sthita-dhīḥ kim prabhāṣheta kim āsīta vrajeta kim || BG 2.54||

arjuna uvācha—Arjun said; **sthita-prajñasya**—one with steady intellect; **kā**—what; **bhāṣhā**—talk; **samādhi-sthasya**—situated in divine consciousness; **Keshava**—Shree Krishna, killer of the Keshi Demon; **sthita-dhīḥ**—enlightened person; **kim**—what; **prabhāṣheta**—talks; **kim**—how; **āsīta**—sits; **vrajeta**—walks; **kim**—how

Meaning- Arjun said: O Keshav, what is the disposition of one who is situated in divine consciousness? How does an enlightened person talk? How does he sit? How does he walk?

śhrī bhagavān uvācha

prajahāti yadā kāmān sarvān pārtha mano-gatān

ātmany-evātmanā tuṣhṭaḥ sthita-prajñas tadochyate || BG 2.55||

śhrī-bhagavān uvācha—The Supreme Lord said; **prajahāti**—discards; **yadā**—when; **kāmān**—selfish desires; **sarvān**—all; **pārtha**—Arjun, the son of Pritha; **manaḥ-gatān**—of the mind; **ātmani**—of the self; **eva**—only; **ātmanā**—by the purified mind; **tuṣhṭaḥ**—satisfied; **sthita-prajñaḥ**—one with steady intellect; **tadā**—at that time; **uchyate**—is said

Meaning- The Supreme Lord said: O Parth when one discards all selfish desires and cravings of the senses that torment the mind, and becomes satisfied in the realization of the self, such a person is said to be transcendentally situated.

duḥkheṣhv-anudvigna-manāḥ sukheṣhu vigata-spṛihaḥ

vīta-rāga-bhaya-krodhaḥ sthita-dhīr munir uchyate || BG 2.56||

duḥkheṣhu—amidst miseries; **anudvigna-manāḥ**—one whose mind is undisturbed; **sukheṣhu**—in pleasure; **vigata-spṛihaḥ**—without craving; **vīta**—free from; **rāga**—attachment; **bhaya**—fear; **krodhaḥ**—anger; **sthita-dhīḥ**—enlightened person; **muniḥ**—a sage; **uchyate**—is called

Meaning- One whose mind remains undisturbed amidst misery, who does not crave pleasure, and who is free from attachment, fear, and anger, is called a sage of steady wisdom.

yaḥ sarvatr-ānabhisnehas tat tat prāpya śhubhāśhubham

nābhi-nandati na dveṣhṭi tasya prajñā pratiṣhṭhitā || BG 2.57||

yaḥ—who; **sarvatra**—in all conditions; **anabhisnehaḥ**—unattached; **tat**—that; **tat**—that; **prāpya**—attaining; **śubha**—good; **aśhubham**—evil; **na**—neither; **abhinandati**—delight in; **na**—nor; **dveṣhṭi**—dejected by; **tasya**—his; **prajñā**—knowledge; **pratiṣhṭhitā**—is fixed

Meaning- One who remains unattached under all conditions, and is neither delighted by good fortune nor dejected by tribulation, is a sage with perfect knowledge.

yadā sanharate chāyaṁ kūrmo' ṅgānīva sarvaśhaḥ

indriyāṇīndriyārthebhyas tasya prajñā pratiṣhṭhitā || BG 2.58||

yadā—when; **sanharate**—withdraw; **cha**—and; **ayam**—this; **kūrmaḥ**—tortoise; **aṅgāni**—limbs; **iva**—as; **sarvaśhaḥ**—fully; **indriyāṇi**—senses; **indriya-arthebhyaḥ**—from the sense objects; **tasya**—his; **prajñā**—divine wisdom; **pratiṣhṭhitā**—fixed in

Meaning- One who can withdraw the senses from their objects, just as a tortoise withdraws its limbs into its shell, is established in divine wisdom.

viṣhayā vinivartante nirāhārasya dehinaḥ

rasa-varjaṁ raso 'pyasya paraṁ dṛiṣhṭvā nivartate || BG 2.59||

viṣhayāḥ—objects for senses; **vinivartante**—restrain; **nirāhārasya**—practicing self-restraint; **dehinaḥ**—for the embodied; **rasa-varjam**—cessation of taste; **rasaḥ**—taste; **api**—however; **asya**—person's; **param**—the Supreme; **dṛiṣhṭvā**—on realization; **nivartate**—ceases to be

Meaning- Aspirants may restrain the senses from their objects of enjoyment, but the taste for the sense objects remains. However, even this taste ceases for those who realize the Supreme.

yatato hyapi kaunteya puruṣhasya vipaśhchitaḥ

indriyāṇi pramāthīni haranti prasabhaṁ manaḥ || BG 2.60||

yatataḥ—while practicing self-control; **hi**—for; **api**—even; **kaunteya**—Arjun, the son of Kunti; **puruṣhasya**—of a person; **vipaśhchitaḥ**—one endowed with discrimination; **indriyāṇi**—the senses; **pramāthīni**—turbulent; **haranti**—carry away; **prasabham**—forcibly; **manaḥ**—the mind

Meaning- The senses are so strong and turbulent, O son of Kunti, that they can forcibly carry away the mind even of a person endowed with discrimination who practices self-control.

tāni sarvāṇi sanyamya yukta āsīta mat-paraḥ

vaśhe hi yasyendriyāṇi tasya prajñā pratiṣhṭhitā || BG 2.61||

tāni—them; **sarvāṇi**—all; **sanyamya**—subduing; **yuktaḥ**—united; **āsīta**—seated; **mat-paraḥ**—toward me (Shree Krishna); **vaśhe**—control; **hi**—certainly; **yasya**—whose; **indriyāṇi**—senses; **tasya**—their; **prajñā**—perfect knowledge; **pratiṣhṭhitā**—is fixed;

Meaning- They are established in perfect knowledge, who subdue their senses and keep their minds ever absorbed in Me.

dhyāyato viṣhayān puṁsaḥ saṅgas teṣhūpajāyate

saṅgāt sañjāyate kāmaḥ kāmāt krodho 'bhijāyate || BG 2.62||

dhyāyataḥ—contemplating; **viṣhayān**—sense objects; **puṁsaḥ**—of a person; **saṅgaḥ**—attachment; **teṣhu**—to them (sense objects); **upajāyate**—arises; **saṅgāt**—from attachment; **sañjāyate**—develops; **kāmaḥ**—desire; **kāmāt**—from desire; **krodhaḥ**—anger; **abhijāyate**—arises

Meaning- While contemplating the objects of the senses, one develops an attachment to them. Attachment leads to desire, and from desire arises anger.

krodhād bhavati sammohaḥ sammohāt smṛiti-vibhramaḥ

smṛiti-bhranśhād buddhi-nāśho buddhi-nāśhāt praṇaśhyati

|| BG 2.63||

krodhāt—from anger; **bhavati**—comes; **sammohaḥ**—clouding of judgement; **sammohāt**—from clouding of judgement; **smṛiti**—memory; **vibhramaḥ**—bewilderment; **smṛiti-bhranśhāt**—from bewilderment of memory; **buddhi-nāśhaḥ**—destruction of intellect; **buddhi-nāśhāt**—from destruction of intellect; **praṇaśhyati**—one is ruined

Meaning- Anger leads to clouding of judgment, which results in bewilderment of memory. When memory is bewildered, the intellect gets destroyed; and when the intellect is destroyed, one is ruined.

rāga-dveṣha-viyuktais tu viṣhayān indriyaiśh charan

ātma-vaśhyair-vidheyātmā prasādam adhigachchhati || BG 2.64||

rāga—attachment; **dveṣha**—aversion; **viyuktaiḥ**—free; **tu**—but; **viṣhayān**—objects of the senses; **indriyaiḥ**—by the senses;

charan—while using; **ātma-vaśhyaiḥ**—controlling one's mind; **vidheya-ātmā**—one who controls the mind; **prasādam**—grace of God; **adhigachchhati**—attains

Meaning- But one who controls the mind, and is free from attachment and aversion, even while using the objects of the senses, attains the Grace of God.

prasāde sarva-duḥkhānāṁ hānir asyopajāyate

prasanna-chetaso hyāśhu buddhiḥ paryavatiṣhṭhate || BG 2.65||

prasāde—by divine grace; **sarva**—all; **duḥkhānām**—sorrows; **hāniḥ**—destruction; **asya**—his; **upajāyate**—comes; **prasanna-chetasaḥ**—with a tranquil mind; **hi**—indeed; **āśhu**—soon; **buddhiḥ**—intellect; **paryavatiṣhṭhate**—becomes firmly established

Meaning- By divine grace comes the peace in which all sorrows end and the intellect of such a person of tranquil mind soon becomes firmly established in God.

nāsti buddhir-ayuktasya na chāyuktasya bhāvanā

na chābhāvayataḥ śhāntir aśhāntasya kutaḥ sukham || BG 2.66||

na—not; **asti**—is; **buddhiḥ**—intellect; **ayuktasya**—not united; **na**—not; **cha**—and; **ayuktasya**—not united; **bhāvanā**—contemplation; **na**—nor; **cha**—and; **abhāvayataḥ**—for those not united; **śhāntiḥ**—peace; **aśhāntasya**—of the unpeaceful; **kutaḥ**—where; **sukham**—happiness

Meaning- But an undisciplined person, who has not controlled the mind and senses, can neither have a resolute intellect nor steady contemplation on God. For one who never unites the mind with God there is no peace; and how can one who lacks peace be happy?

tasmād yasya mahā-bāho nigṛihītāni sarvaśhaḥ

indriyāṇīndriyārthebhyas tasya prajñā pratiṣhṭhitā || BG 2.68||

tasmāt—therefore; **yasya**—whose; **mahā-bāho**—mighty-armed one; **nigṛihītāni**—restrained; **sarvaśhaḥ**—completely; **indriyāṇi**—senses; **indriya-arthebhyaḥ**—from sense objects; **tasya**—of that person; **prajñā**—transcendental knowledge; **pratiṣhṭhitā**—remains fixed

Meaning- Therefore, one who has restrained the senses from their objects, O mighty-armed Arjun, is firmly established in transcendental knowledge.

Concept Of Bhakti Yoga-

Complete love and devotion towards the supreme are referred to as **Bhakti**. This concept is discussed extensively in Chapter 12 of the Bhagavad Gita.

arjuna uvācha

evaṁ satata-yuktā ye bhaktās tvāṁ paryupāsate

ye chāpy akṣharam avyaktaṁ teṣhāṁ ke yoga-vittamāḥ ||BG 12.1||

arjunaḥ uvācha—Arjun said; **evam**—thus; **satata**—steadfastly; **yuktāḥ**—devoted; **ye**—those; **bhaktāḥ**—devotees; **tvām**—you; **paryupāsate**—worship; **ye**—those; **cha**—and; **api**—also; **akṣharam**—the imperishable; **avyaktam**—the formless Brahman; **teṣhām**—of them; **ke**—who; **yoga-vit-tamāḥ**—more perfect in Yog

Meaning- Arjun inquired: Between those who are steadfastly devoted to Your personal form and those who worship the formless Brahman, whom do You consider to be more perfect in Yog?

śhrī-bhagavān uvācha

mayy āveśhya mano ye māṁ nitya-yuktā upāsate

śhraddhayā parayopetās te me yuktatamā matāḥ || BG 12.2||

śhrī-bhagavān uvācha—the Lord said; **mayi**—on Me; **āveśhya**—fix; **manaḥ**—the mind; **ye**—those; **mām**—Me; **nitya yuktāḥ**—always engaged; **upāsate**—worship; **śhraddhayā**—with faith; **parayā**—best; **upetāḥ**—endowed; **te**—they; **me**—by Me; **yukta-tamāḥ**—situated highest in Yog; **matāḥ**—I consider

Meaning- The Lord said: Those who fix their minds on Me and always engage in My devotion with steadfast faith, I consider them to be the best yogis.

ye tv akṣharam anirdeśhyam avyaktaṁ paryupāsate

sarvatra-gam achintyañcha kūṭa-stham achalandhruvam

||BG 12.3||

sanniyamyendriya-grāmaṁ sarvatra sama-buddhayaḥ

te prāpnuvanti mām eva sarva-bhūta-hite ratāḥ ||BG 12.4||

ye—who; **tu**—but; **akṣharam**—the imperishable; **anirdeśhyam**—the indefinable; **avyaktam**—the unmanifest; **paryupāsate**—worship; **sarvatra-gam**—the all-pervading; **achintyam**—the unthinkable; **cha**—and; **kūṭa-stham**—the unchanging; **achalam**—the immovable; **dhruvam**—the eternal.

sanniyamya—restraining; **indriya-grāmam**—the senses; **sarvatra**—everywhere; **sama-buddhayaḥ**—even-minded; **te**—they; **prāpnuvanti**—attain; **mām**—Me; **eva**—also; **sarva-bhūta-hite**—in the welfare of all beings; **ratāḥ**—engaged

<u>Meaning</u> - But those who worship the formless aspect of the Absolute Truth—the imperishable, the indefinable, the unmanifest, the all-pervading, the unthinkable, the unchanging, the eternal, and the immoveable—by restraining their senses and being even-minded everywhere, such persons, engaged in the welfare of all beings, also attain Me.

Concept Of Karma Yoga-

Discussion on Action remains the core theme of the Bhagavad Gita. This concept has been mentioned time and again in various chapters as Shri Krishan considers **renouncing the fruits of action** to be the highest quality. In chapter 3, titled **Karma Yoga**, Krishna discusses this concept in detail. The same concept is discussed in Chapter 2, titled **Samkhya Yoga.**

karmaṇy-evādhikāras te mā phaleṣhu kadāchana

mā karma-phala-hetur bhūr mā te saṅgo 'stvakarmaṇi ||BG 2.47||

Introduction To Yoga Text

karmaṇi—in prescribed duties; **Eva**—only; **adhikāraḥ**—right; **te**—your; **mā**—not; **phaleṣhu**—in the fruits; **kadāchana**—at any time; **mā**—never; **karma-phala**—results of the activities; **hetuḥ**—cause; **bhūḥ**—be; **mā**—not; **te**—your; **saṅgaḥ**—attachment; **astu**—must be; **akarmaṇi**—in inaction

Meaning- You have a right to perform your prescribed duties, but you are not entitled to the fruits of your actions. Never consider yourself to be the cause of the results of your activities, nor be attached to inaction.

yoga-sthaḥ kuru karmāṇi saṅgaṁ tyaktvā dhanañjaya

siddhy-asiddhyoḥ samo bhūtvā samatvaṁ yoga uchyate ||BG 2.48||

yoga-sthaḥ—being steadfast in yog; **kuru**—perform; **karmāṇi**—duties; **saṅgam**—attachment; **tyaktvā**—having abandoned; **dhanañjaya**—Arjun; **siddhi-asiddhyoḥ**—in success and failure; **samaḥ**—equipoised; **bhūtvā**—becoming; **samatvam**—equanimity; **yogaḥ**—Yog; **uchyate**—is called

Meaning - Be steadfast in the performance of your duty, O Arjun, abandoning attachment to success and failure. Such equanimity is called Yog.

dūreṇa hy-avaraṁ karma buddhi-yogād dhanañjaya

buddhau śharaṇam anvichchha kṛipaṇāḥ phala-hetavaḥ || BG 2.49||

dūreṇa—(discard) from far away; **hi**—certainly; **avaram**—inferior; **karma**—reward-seeking actions; **buddhi-yogāt**—with the intellect established in Divine knowledge; **dhanañjaya**—Arjun;

buddhau—divine knowledge and insight; **sharaṇam**—refuge; **anvichchha**—seek; **kṛipaṇāḥ**—miserly; **phala-hetavaḥ**—those seeking fruits of their work

Meaning - Seek refuge in divine knowledge and insight, O Arjun, and discard reward-seeking actions that are certainly inferior to works performed with the intellect established in Divine knowledge. Miserly are those who seek to enjoy the fruits of their works.

buddhi-yukto jahātīha ubhe sukṛita-duṣhkṛite

tasmād yogāya yujyasva yogaḥ karmasu kauśhalam ||BG 2.50||

buddhi-yuktaḥ—endowed with wisdom; **jahāti**—get rid of; **iha**—in this life; **ubhe**—both; **sukṛita-duṣhkṛite**—good and bad deeds; **tasmāt**—therefore; **yogāya**—for Yog; **yujyasva**—strive for; **yogaḥ**—yog is; **karmasu kauśhalam**—the art of working skilfully

Meaning - One who prudently practices the science of work without attachment can get rid of both good and bad reactions in this life itself. Therefore, strive for Yog, which is **Skill in Action**.

<u>**Concept Of Dhyana Yoga**</u> - Shri Krishan explains Dhyan Yog as constant meditation on to the supreme with a disciplined mind. **Chapter 6** has a detailed discussion of techniques, paths, and consequences of Dhyan Yog.

ārurukṣhor muner yogaṁ karma kāraṇam uchyate

yogārūḍhasya tasyaiva śhamaḥ kāraṇam uchyate ||BG 6.3||

ārurukṣhoḥ—a beginner; **muneḥ**—of a sage; **yogam**—Yog; **karma**—working without attachment; **kāraṇam**—the cause;

uchyate—is said; **yoga ārūḍhasya**—of those who are elevated in Yog; **tasya**—their; **eva**—certainly; **śhamaḥ**—meditation; **kāraṇam**—the cause; **uchyate**—is said

<u>Meaning</u> - To the soul who is aspiring for perfection in Yog, work without attachment is said to be the means; to the sage who is already elevated in Yog, tranquillity in meditation is said to be the means.

śhuchau deśhe pratiṣhṭhāpya sthiram āsanam ātmanaḥ

nātyuchchhritaṁ nāti-nīchaṁ chailājina-kuśhottaram ||BG 6.11||

śhuchau—in a clean; **deśhe**—place; **pratiṣhṭhāpya**—having established; **sthiram**—steadfast; **āsanam**—seat; **ātmanaḥ**—his own; **na**—not; **ati**—too; **uchchhritam**—high; **na**—not; **ati**—too; **nīcham**—low; **chaila**—cloth; **ajina**—a deerskin; **kuśha**—Kuśh grass; **uttaram**—one over the other

<u>Meaning</u> - To practice Yog, one should make an āsan (seat) in a sanctified place, by placing Kuśh grass, deerskin, and a cloth, one over the other. The āsan should be neither too high nor too low.

tatraikāgraṁ manaḥ kṛitvā yata-chittendriya-kriyaḥ

upaviśhyāsane yuñjyād yogam ātma-viśhuddhaye ||BG 6.12||

samaṁ kāya-śhiro-grīvaṁ dhārayann achalaṁ sthiraḥ

samprekṣhya nāsikāgraṁ svaṁ diśhaśh chānavalokayan ||BG 6.13||

tatra—there; **eka-agram**—one-pointed; **manaḥ**—mind; **kṛitvā**—having made; **yata-chitta**—controlling the mind;

indriya—senses; **kriyaḥ**—activities; **upaviśhya**—being seated; **āsane**—on the seat; **yuñjyāt yogam**—should strive to practice yog; **ātma viśhuddhaye**—for purification of the mind;

samam—straight; **kāya**—body; **śhiraḥ**—head; **grīvam**—neck; **dhārayan**—holding; **achalam**—unmoving; **sthiraḥ**—still; **samprekṣhya**—gazing; **nāsika-agram**—at the tip of the nose; **svam**—own; **diśhaḥ**—directions; **cha**—and; **anavalokayan**—not looking

<u>Meaning</u> - Seated firmly on it, the yogi should strive to purify the mind by focusing it in meditation with one-pointed concentration, controlling all thoughts activities. He must hold the body, neck, and head firmly in a straight line, and gaze at the tip of the nose, without allowing the eyes to wander.

praśhāntātmā vigata-bhīr brahmachāri-vrate sthitaḥ

manaḥ sanyamya mach-chitto yukta āsīta mat-paraḥ ||BG 6.15||

praśhānta—serene; **ātmā**—mind; **vigata-bhīḥ**—fearless; **brahmachāri-vrate**—in the vow of celibacy; **sthitaḥ**—situated; **manaḥ**—mind; **sanyamya**—having controlled; **mat-chittaḥ**—meditate on me (Shree Krishna); **yuktaḥ**—engaged; **āsīta**—should sit; **mat-paraḥ**—having me as the supreme goal

Meaning- Thus, with a serene, fearless, and unwavering mind, and staunch in the vow of celibacy, the vigilant yogi should meditate on Me, having Me alone as the supreme goal.

Significance of Bhagavad Gita in day-to-day life

Bhagwad Gita is part of Mahabharat. This great text is a conversation between Shri Krishna and Arjuna. **It has 18 chapters and 700 shlokas.** It offers a very practical approach to life. It takes us to the root of the problems/miseries in our lives and suggests ways to handle the fundamental cause of these problems.

- Gita clearly puts the law of karma as the basis of everything that happens in human life. And then offers a way in the form of "Getting detached from the fruits of action" in order to cut the cycle of the law of karma.
- Teachings like **Samatvam Yog Uchyate (Being equanimous), Yogah Karmashu Kauśhalam (Skill in action), Yukta-Ahara-Vihārasya (moderate eating & recreation), Ma Phaleṣhu Kadāchana (No rights on the fruits of the action), etc.** are very crucial for a healthy and happy life.
- If one understands and adapts any of the 4 concepts mentioned in the Bhagwad Gita, **Karma Yoga, Bhakti Yoga, Dhyana Yoga, and Jnana Yoga,** then one can easily get rid of mental stress.
- Gita clearly tells us to stick to our own duties (Dharma), rather than doing someone else's duties. Adapting just this one concept can give clarity as well as the liberation of the mind.
- Gita suggests ways to get rid of the fears in life. It also clearly points out that anger (Krodha) is the very reason people make incorrect choices which will eventually lead to the downfall of a person.

All of the above-mentioned teachings are just the tip of the iceberg. The entire 18 chapters are full of such pearls which have been and will always be significant for living a balanced life

Concept of healthy living in Bhagavad Gita (Ahara, Vihara, Achara, Vichara)

Bhagwad Gits specifies that **moderation** is the key principle of healthy living. It suggests applying moderation in all aspects of life such as-

- Yukta - Ahara (Moderate - food)
- Yukta - Vihara (Moderate - recreation),
- Yukta - Achara (Moderate - conduct),
- Yukta - Vichara (Moderate - thinking),

These principles guide the practitioner to bring reforms in their lifestyle to overcome irregularities in their routine life.

yuktāhāra-vihārasya yukta-cheṣhṭasya karmasu

yukta-svapnāvabodhasya yogo bhavati duḥkha-hā ||BG 6.17||

yukta—moderate; **āhāra**—eating; **vihārasya**—recreation; **yukta cheṣhṭasya karmasu**—balanced in work; **yukta**—regulated; **svapna-avabodhasya**—sleep and wakefulness; **yogaḥ**—Yog; **bhavati**—becomes; **duḥkha-hā**—the slayer of sorrows

<u>Meaning</u>- But those who are temperate in eating and recreation, balanced in work, and regulated in sleep, can mitigate all sorrows by practicing Yog.

2.4 Study of Patanjali Yoga Sutra

Including selected sutras from the following chapters- (Chapters 1- 1 to 12, Chapters 2 - 46 to 51, Chapters 3 - 1 to 4).

Imp - All of these Sutras need to be memorized with the meaning as these will be asked in the practical exam.

Chapter – 1 Samadhi Pada (1-12)

Atha yoga-anuśāsanam ||PYS1.1||

Atha - now, **Yoga** - yog, **Anuśāsanam** - the discipline begins.

Meaning - Now, the yogic discipline begins.

yogaś-chitta-vṛtti-nirodhaḥ ||PYS 1.2||

Yogas - Yog (is), **Chitta** - mind-stuff, **Vritti** - fluctuations (of mind),

Nirodhah - restrain

Meaning- The complete cessation of fluctuation of mind is Yoga.

tadā draṣṭuḥ svarūpe-'vasthānam ||PYS 1.3||

tada - at that time, **drashtuh** - the seer, **avasthanam** - rests, remaining,

Swaroop - in His own nature

Meaning- At that time (When the mental fluctuations are restrained) the seer (the self) remains in his own nature,

vṛtti sārūpyam-itaratra ||PYS 1.4||

vritti - modification, **sarupyam** - identification, **itaratra** - at other times

Meaning- At other times (When the mind is full of fluctuation), when not in the state of yoga the seer (the self) is identified with the modification.

vṛttayaḥ pañcatayyaḥ kliṣṭākliṣṭāḥ ||PYS 1.5||

vrittayah - the modifications, **panchatayyah** - five kinds, **klishta** - painful, **aklishta** - not painful

Meaning- There are five kinds of mental modification (vritti) which are either painful or not painful. Any information which the mind receives causes some kind of waves in the mind. Such as-

- Eating your favourite food causes a pleasant wave (Aklishta Vritti), and misunderstanding rope as a snake causes a wave of fear in the mind (klishta Vritti).
- Receiving the news of a death will cause unpleasant / Klishta Vrittis in Chitta, whereas receiving the news of birth will cause pleasant / Aklishta Vrittis in Chitta.

pramāṇa viparyaya vikalpa nidrā smṛtayaḥ ||PYS 1.6||

pramana - Right Knowledge, **viparyaya** – indiscrimination / false knowledge, **vikalpa** – misconception/fantasy, **nidra** - sleep, **smritayah** – memory

Meaning- They are – Pramana, Viparyaya, Vikalpa, Nidra, Smriti.

pratyakṣa-anumāna-āgamāḥ pramāṇāni ||PYS 1.7||

pratyaksha - Perception, **anumana** - Inference, **agamah** - competent evidence, **pramanani** - sources of right knowledge.

Meaning- Pramana Vritti (Right knowledge) can further be divided into Pratyaksha (Perception), Anumana (Inference), and Agama (competent evidence).

- Any information which you experience yourself such as seeing the fire with your own eyes is termed Pratyaksha Vritti.
- You see the smoke far away and you infer that there must be fire is referred to as Anumana Vritti.
- Someone you trust tells you that there is a fire and you choose to believe that person, this is referred to as Agama Vritti.

The fluctuations caused in the mind through this perceived knowledge can either be pleasant (Aklishta) or unpleasant (Aklishta).

viparyayo mithyā-jñānam-atadrūpa pratiṣṭham ||PYS 1.8||

viparyaya - indiscrimination, wrong knowledge, **mithya** - false, illusory, **jnanam** - knowledge, **atadroopa** - not its own nature, **pratishtham** -based on, established

Meaning- Viparyaya Vritti is considered false knowledge that is not based on the real nature of its object. For instance- Believing in rumors or flattery, misunderstanding rope as a snake, etc.

śabda-jñāna-anupātī vastu-śūnyo vikalpaḥ ||PYS 1.9||

shabda - verbal, **jnana** - knowledge, cognition, **anupati** - following, arises, proceed, **Vastu** - reality, **shoonyo** - empty, devoid, **vikalpa** - imagination, fantasy, verbal misconception.

Meaning- Vikalpa arises from verbal cognition that is devoid of reality. It can be simply understood as fantasy or imagination. Something which is only happening in the mind.

For instance- The habit of creating different scenarios in the mind and indulging in them up to the point of avoiding reality can be an example of extreme Vikalpa Vritti.

abhāva pratyayālambanā vṛttirnidrā ||PYS 1.10||

abhava - non-existence, voidness, **pratyaya** - mental state, feeling, **alambana** - based, support, **vritti** - modification, various forms of the mind-field, **Nidra** - deep sleep

Meaning- Nidra (Deep sleep) is the absence of all impressions or it is a feeling of voidness.

This sutra is actually **pretty intriguing.** What kind of fluctuations can Nidra cause in the mind? What happens when you sleep? Also, if there are no dreams then the mind is also devoid of impressions of outside experiences.

And most importantly why is this a vritti?

This may be the **hardest Vritti** to understand as there is no way for us to know what happens when we sleep. All we remember is that we slept well or we didn't sleep well. If you look at the mind field/ Chitta as a screen on which all the Vrittis can be projected, Then Nidra would be a state where there is just a black slide on the screen.

Though you won't see anything on the slide, meaning you won't remember anything from the sleep but it is still a projection on the Chitta.

Another way to look at it is that nidra can actually be a hindrance to spiritual progress. Imagine sitting in meditation and falling asleep. Or sleeping in Shavasana.

We need to avoid this tendency so we can deepen the meditation experience. Now, with this understanding of the Nidra and the unconscious impression it leaves on the mind, we can find ways to bring this Vritti under conscious control, like all the other four kinds of Vrittis. And it also means that we will have to go beyond Nidra to find the Self.

Just like other Vrittis, Nidra is also Klishta or Aklishta. Sleeping for that much duration when the body quickly gets rested and restores the rejuvenations can be termed as Aklishta nidra Vriti but on the other hand, someone who is excessively dominant by Nidra Vritti and sleeps the whole day, would you call that person a spiritually inclined person, or in practical terms would that person be able to accomplish anything? Hence Klishta Nidra Vritti.

Another commonly asked question is **"What is the difference between Nidra and Samadhi?"** The simple answer could be that Nidra is an unconscious process, whereas Samadhi is a conscious sadhana.

anu-bhūta-viṣaya-asaṁpramoṣaḥ smṛtiḥ ||PYS 1.11||

anubhoota - experienced, **vishaya** – object / impressions,

asampramoshah - not being stolen, **smriti** - memory, remembering

Meaning- Smriti is the vritti when once-perceived objects are not forgotten and keep coming back to the consciousness. Such as thinking about the time when you won a prize gives a pleasant fluctuation in the mind, hence Aklishta Smriti Vritti, and thinking about a painful time gives a rather unpleasant fluctuation in the mind hence Klishta Smriti Vritti.

abhyāsa vairāgyābhyām tannirōdhaḥ ||PYS 1.12||

abhyasa - repeated practice, **vairagyabhyam** - non-attachment, **tat** - of those/ these, **nirodhah** - control

Meaning- Repeated practice and dispassion/detachment are the means to stop the modifications of the mind.

There is no mention of which particular practice is he referring to. But it is understood to be the practice of Ashtanga Yoga. An integrated approach of practicing social and personal disciplines (Yamas and Niyama), a healthy diet, asana, pranayama, and meditation regularly with an attitude of letting go of the attachment and aversions both, will help to control the Vrittis.

It's important to notice that Patanjali doesn't say to control only the Aklishta vritti. **This is in line with the core concept of Santana Culture, "To be able to stay balanced in unpleasant as well as pleasant situations".**

Chapter 2- Sadhana Pada (46-51)

Sthira-sukham-asanam ||PYS 2.46||

sthira - steady / firm, **sukham** - pleasant, **asanam** - posture

Meaning- Asana (Posture) is that which is steady and pleasant

Prayatna--shaithilya-ananta-samapattibhyam ||PYS 2.47||

Prayatna - effort, **Shaithilya** - relaxation, **Ananta** - infinite,

Samapattibhyam - by focusing / by meditating.

Meaning- In order to achieve that (Sthiram-Sukham-Asanam) one should do relaxed efforts with an intent focus on the supreme.

The word **"Relaxed Effort"** is significant here. Asana practice should be done with absolute ease. The opening of the joints and muscles takes time, one should learn to be patient with oneself.

Tato-dvandva-anabhighatah ||PYS 2.48||

tatah - then, **dvandva** - the dualities, **anabhighatah** - being beyond disturbance.

Meaning- Once the asana is firmed, one is undisturbed by the dualities.

This sutra talks about staying balanced irrespective of the situation. Patanjali says that Asana practice can also help in achieving this balanced state. Meaning, staying balanced in heat or cold, pleasure or pain, happiness or sadness, success or failure, etc.

Tasmin-satishvasa-prashvasayor-gativichchhedah-pranayamah ||PYS 2.49||

Tasmin - in this, **sati** - being accomplished, **shvasa** - inhalation, **prashvasayo** - exhalation, **gati** - flow, **vichchhedah** - cessation, **pranayamah** - breath regulation, pranayama.

Meaning- Controlling the motion of the inhalation and the exhalation once this (asana) is accomplished is Pranayama.

bahya-abhyantara-stambha vrittih-desha-kala-sankhyabhih-paridrishto-dirgha-sookshmah ||PYS 2.50||

bahya - external, **abhyantara** - internal, **stambha** - motionless, **vrittih** - modifications, **desha** - place, **kala** - time, **sankhyabhih** - number, **paridrishto** - regulated, **dirgha** - long, **sookshmah** - subtle.

Meaning- The pranayama has external, internal, or motionless modifications. They are to be regulated by place (different sections in the body such as the clavicular, thoracic, or abdomen), time (Duration), and number (counts). Pranayama can be either long or short.

bahya-abhyantara-vishaya-akshepi-chaturthah ||PYS 2.51||

bahya - external, **abhyantara** - internal, **vishaya** - objective, **akshepi** – transcending, **chaturthah** - the fourth.

Meaning- The fourth pranayama is restraining the prana directing it either externally or internally.

This is also referred to as **Kevala Kumbhaka** in Hatha Yoga.

Chapter 3- Vibhuti Pada (1 to 4)

Desha-bandhash-chittasya-dharana ||PYS 3.1||

desha - point/object, **bandha** – holding/fixation, **chittasya** – mind/consciousness, **dharana** - concentration.

Meaning- Dharana is holding the mind to one place /object /or point.

tatra pratyayaikatanata dhyanam ||PYS 3.2||

tatra - in that, **pratyaya** - mental modifications, **ikatanata** - continuous flow of similar, **dhyanam** - meditation.

Meaning- In that (Dharana) the unbroken flow of similar mental modifications is called Dhyana.

tad evarthamatranirbhasam svaroopashoonyam iva samadhih ||PYS 3.3||

tad - that, **eva** - as it were, **artha** - object, **matra** - only, **nirbhasam** - shining, **sva** - own, **roopa** - form, **shoonyam** - empty, **devoid**- is absent, **iva** – like/ as it were, **samadhih** - oneness, integration.

Meaning- Samadhi is when the object of meditation only shines forth, as though devoid of its own form.

trayam ekatra sanyamah ||PYS 3.4||

trayam - the three, **ekatra** - together, **sanyamah** - samyama.

Meaning- The three (Dharana, Dhyana, and Samadhi) together on the same object are called **Samyama**

2.5 Important Concept in Patanjali Yoga Sutra

Chitta

Chitta can be understood as a section of the mind where all the impressions of the outside world are stored. It is also termed mind-stuff or mind-field. Patanjali says that **fluctuations (Vritti)** in the Chitta are the **main reason** for misery/unhappiness in human beings. That is why he gives the meaning of Yoga as "Chitta-vritti-nirodhah", meaning "To stop the fluctuation in the mind is Yoga."

Apart from Patanjali Yog Sutra, the reference to "Chitta" is found in several other texts. Such as-

The Upanishads explain Chitta as part of **Antahkarana Chatushtaya**. Antahkarana Chatushtaya is a term that is collectively used for 4 different faculties of mind- **Chitta**- Storehouse of samskara/impressions, **Buddhi**- Decision-making faculty, **Manas**- Synthesizing faculty, **Ahamkara**- The Ego, I-am-ness

However, **Samkhya philosophy** says that the Antahkarana refers to only 3 faculties- **Buddhi, Manas, Ahamkara**.

Here there is **no mention of Chitta**. This indicates that as per Samkhya Darshan the term "Buddhi" serves two purposes- Decision-making faculty, and A storehouse of samskara/impressions.

Now, In the **Patanjali Yoga Sutra**, there is **no mention of Buddhi**, therefore we may consider the term Chitta used by Patanjali to be the same as the term Buddhi of Sankhya. In Patanjali Yog Sutra the Antahkarana is comprised of- **Chitta, Manas, Ahamkara**.

Chitta Vritti- (Refer to chapter 2.4 for detailed information on vritti)

Chitta-vritti-nirodhah-upaya - The solutions to control the modifications of the mind.

Abhyasa-Vairagyabhyam-tan-nirodhah ||PYS 1.12||

(Refer to Chapter 2.4 for the explanation of this sutra)

As we read the Patanjali Yog Sutra further, we came across various practices mentioned by Patanjali-

1. **Ishwara Pranidhana-** Surrender to the supreme
2. **Chitta Prasadana-** 4 different attitudes towards 4 different kinds of people.
3. **The practice of Bahya Kumbhaka-** He says the mind can also be calmed down with retention of breath after forceful exhalation
4. **Pratipaksha Bhavana-** The practice of holding thoughts of an opposite nature. Such as when the idea of hinsa (violence) comes, then thoughts of non-violence should be brought to mind. When the idea of hate comes then the thoughts of love and compassion should be brought to mind.
5. **Ashtanga Yoga-** This is an 8-limbed practice of achieving the Liberation.

We should take note of Patanjali's advice of **"Ektattva Abhyasa"**, meaning whichever practice we choose we should stick to it diligently.

Kleshas

Kleshas are what generate pain in our experience. There are 5 Kleshas that would come with the Vrittis- **Avidya (Ignorance), Asmita (Egoism), Raga (Attachment), Dvesha (Aversion), Abhinivesha (Clinging to life/ Fear of death).**

Of these five, **"Avidya"** (ignorance) is the **mother of all the Kleshas**. Kleshas manifest in human beings in **four degrees-** Prasupta (Dormant), Tanu (Weak), Vichhina (Oscillating), and Udara (Abundant).

Our objective is to bring the klesha from the Udara(abundant) state to Vichhina (Oscillating), then from Vichhina to Tanu (Weak), and from there to the Prasupta (Dormant) state.

Kriya Yog helps in bringing the Kleshas to a weak or "Tanu" state.

tapah-svadhyaya-ishvara-pranidhanani-kriyayogah ||2.1||

Meaning - Austerity, the study of sacred literature, and complete surrender to the supreme, these 3 practices are collectively called **Kriya-Yoga.**

Do not get confused with the same being mentioned as part of Niyama. These 3 are mentioned separately as well and referred to as Kriya Yoga.

It is important to understand that **Ishwara** here does not refer to a personal deity, instead, it is one universal power, referred to as **"Purusha Vishesha / Supreme Self". Patanjali does not mention any ritual, rites, or, worship towards "Ishwara".** Hence Ishwara in Patanjali's Yoga Sutra is not a religious/personal

God, and that's why **Yoga is not a religious practice. It's a lifestyle based on one-ness.**

Chitta Bhumi

The theory of Chitta Bhumi originates from Patanjali Yoga Sutra, but it is elaborated in **"Yoga Bhashya"** which is a commentary by sage **Veda Vyasa** on the yoga Sutra. Chitta Bhumi refers to the different planes of the mind. Sage Vyasa speaks about 5 Chitta Bhumis.

Kshiptam Moodham Vikshiptam Ekagram Niruddhamiti Chitta Bhumayah ||Yog Bhashya 1.1||

Kshipta Chitta (The Monkey Mind)- This is dominated by Rajas Guna. This state of mind is restless and roving. Pleasure and pain, like and dislike, love and hate; the monkey mind is always alternating between extreme states.

Moodha Chitta (The donkey mind)- This is dominated by Tamas Guna. Lust, anger, greed, infatuation etc. are the prime traits of the donkey mind. Such Chitta is forgetful, blinded, and possessed of the Nidra vritti. This chitta possesses the least concentration.

Vikshipta Chitta (The Butterfly Mind)- This state oscillates between Satwa and Rajas. Most of us are in a Vikshipta state of mind. Sometimes at complete peace, sometimes anxious, overwhelmed, restless.

Ekagra Chitta (One Pointed Mind)- This is dominated by Sattva. This state of mind is referred to as happy and whole.

Such awakened individuals have single-pointed focus, sharp intuitiveness, and a dissolved ego.

Niruddha (Nirguna / Fully Focused Mind)- This is a transcendental state, referred to as absolute focus or a state of no mind.

The First three mental planes (Chitta Bhumi) are not considered apt for Yoga. But when the mental plane is **Ekagra or Niruddha then Yoga can commence.**

Chitta Vikshepas (Antarayas) and their associates (Sahbhuvas)

Chitta Vikshepas refers to **distractions** of the mind. These are **9 obstacles** during yoga Practice.

Vyadhi (Physical disease), **Styan** (Mental laziness), **Sanshaya** (Doubt), **Pramada** (Carelessness/negligence), **Alasya** (Physical laziness), **Avirati** (Stubborn attachment to sense objects), **Bhranti-Darshan** (False perception), **Alabdha-Bhumikatva** (Failing to attain a firm ground), **Anavasthitattva** (Instability).

These 9 obstacles can be divided into physical, mental, intellectual; and spiritual categories.

Physical- Vyadhi, Alasya, **Mental-** Saṃśhaya, Pramada, Styan, Avirati,

Spiritual- Alabdha Bhumikatva, Anavasthitattva

Sahabhuvas- Patanjali says that these obstacles will be accompanied by their associates, called **"Sahabhuvas"**. 4 **Sahabhuvas** are-

Dukha (Unhappiness), **Daur-manasya** (Despair/depression/frustration), **Angamejayatva** (Tremors in the body), **Svasa-Prasvas** (Erratic breathing pattern)

Patanjali says that Vikshepa-**Sahabhuva** can be removed by **Ek-Tattva- Abhyasa** (Practice of one subject).

Chitta Prasadana

This concept involves taking four different approaches/attitudes towards four different types of people or qualities.

Maitri-Karuna-Mudita-Upekaha-nam- Sukha-Dukha-Punya-Apunya- Vishayanam- Bhavanatah-Chitta - Prasadanam ||PYS 1.33||

maitree -friendship, **karuna** - mercy, **mudita** - gladness, **upekshanam** - indifference, **sukha** - happy, **duhkha** - unhappy, **punya** – good/virtuous, **Apunya** - evil, **Vishayanam** – objects (of experience), **bhavanatah** - by cultivation habits, **Chitta** - mind field/ consciousness, **Prasadanam** - purified.

Meaning

- Maitri (Friendship) with people who are Sukhi (Happy people).
- Karuna(compassion) towards people who are Dukhi (Unhappy people),
- Mudita (Goodwill/happiness) towards people who are Punyatama (Virtuous),
- Upeksha (indifference/ neutral/ equanimous) towards people who are evil or Apunyatma (negative qualities).

Ashtanga Yoga-

yama-niyama-asana-pranayama-pratyahara-dharana-dhyana- samadhayo- ashtauva aṅgāni ||PYS 2.29||

yama - abstinence, **niyama** - observance, **asana** - posture, **pranayama** - breath control, **pratyahara** - sense withdrawal, **dharana** - concentration, **dhyana** - meditation, **samadhyo** - meditation in its higher state, **ashtauva** - eight **aṅgāni** - limbs, parts.

Meaning- Yama, Niyama, Asana, Pranayama, Pratyahara, Dharana, Dhyana, and Samadhi; are the eight limbs of Yoga.

The **first 4 limbs** of Ashtanga Yoga collectively refer to **Bahiranga Yoga** as during these 4 practices the 5 senses are in touch with the outside world. The 5th limb, **Pratyahara** is referred to as the **bridge** between the first 4 limbs (Bahiranga yoga) and the **last 3 limbs (Antaranga yoga)**

Bahiranga Yoga

Yama - Yama refers to the observances and restraints that regulate our interaction with others.

Ahinsā- Satya- Asteya- brahmacharya- Aparigraha- Yamah ||PYS 2.30||

Ahinsa - non-violence, **Satya** - truthfulness, **Asteya** - non-stealing, **brahmacharya** - continence, **Aparigraha** - non-possessiveness/non- greed, **Yamah** – Yama / abstinence

Meaning- Ahimsa, Satya, Asteya, Brahmacharya, and Aparigraha are the five Yamas.

Talking about the importance of the Yamas, Patanjali further says-

Jati-desha-kala-samaya-anavachchhinnah-sarvabhauma-mahavratam ||PYS 2.31||

jati - class, **desha** - place, **kala** - time, **samaya** - circumstance, **ana- vachchhinnah** - universal, **sarva-bhauma** – universal, **mahavratam** - great vow.

Meaning- These Yamas are unbroken by Time, Place, Caste, and Purpose. These are universal vows.

Niyama - Niyama refers to observances and restraints which govern an individual's personal life.

shaucha-santosha-tapah-svadhyaya-eshvara-pranidhanani-niyamah

|| PYS 2.32||

Shaucha – Cleanliness/ internal and external purification, **Santosh** - contentment, **tapaḥ** - austerity, **svādhyāyaḥ** - self-study, **Ishwara- Pranidhanani** – complete devotion/surrender to God, **niyamah** - observances

Meaning- Shaucha, Santosha, Tapa, Swadhayaya, Ishwar Pranidhana are 5 Niyama.

Asana - Patanjali defines asana as-

Sthira-sukham-asanam ||PYS 2.46||

sthira – steady/ firm, **sukham** - pleasant, **asanam** - posture

Meaning- Asana is any state that is stable and pleasant.

Note- Patanjali didn't mention the name of any asana in the whole 195 sutras, he just devotes only 3 sutras for asana. These are Sutra numbers **2.46, 2.47, and 2.48. (Refer to Unit 2.4 for the meaning of these Sutra)**

Pranayama - 4 ways to control the breath are suggested in the yoga Sutra.

Modification of inhalation, Modification of exhalation, Stoppage of breath, and the fourth Pranayama transcends the subject matter of inhalation and exhalation.

Tamsin-sati-shvasa-prashvasa-yor-gati-vichchhedah-pranayamah ||PYS 2.49||

bahya-abhyantara-stambhavrittih-desha-kala-sankhyabhih-paridrishto - dirgha- sookshmah ||2.50||

bahya-abhyantara-vishaya-akshepi-chaturthah ||PYS 2.51|| tataḥ-kṣīyate-prakāśa-āvaraṇam ||PYS 2.52|| dharanasu- cha-yogyata- manasah ||PYS 2.53||

(Refer to Unit 2.4 for the meaning of these Sutra)

Bridge

Pratyahara –

This refers to the withdrawal of sense organs from their respective objects. It is the voluntary withdrawal of sense organs from their respective objects. To understand this better, let's take an example. Has it ever happened to you that you are engaged in some work with such concentration that someone calls your name and you didn't hear it, or when you are listening to some music through earphones and still miss the lyrics? Now, this doesn't happen because we don't have fully functioning ears, but because our mind was focused on someplace else. This is the withdrawal of the sense organ which is "the ear" in this example with the respective object which is "the sound". Pratyahara is the practice of bringing in this withdrawal of senses voluntarily.

sva-vishaya-asamprayoge-chittasya-svarupe-anukarah-iva-indriyanam pratyaharah ||2.54||

tatah-parama-vashyata-indriyanam ||2.55||

(Refer to Unit 2.4 for the meaning of these Sutra)

Antaranga Yoga

Dharana-

Dharana means concentration. Confinement of Chitta to one object is Dharana. In other words, when you sit for mediation and you are trying to concentrate on your object, that process is called Dharana.

deshabandhash-chittasya-dharana ||PYS 3.1||

(Refer to Unit 2.4 for the meaning of these Sutra)

Dhyana –

Dhyana means meditation. In Dharna all the efforts are directed toward keeping distractions away. When these efforts are successful and there are no distractions, the mind reaches the state of "Dhyana". This means, now there is no trying of concentration. Now, you are fully concentrated on the object. As Patanjali explains –

tatra pratyayaikatanata dhyanam ||PYS 3.2||

(Refer to Unit 2.4 for the meaning of these Sutra)

Samadhi

tad evarthamatranirbhasam svaroopashoonyam iva samadhih ||PYS 3.3||

(Refer to Unit 2.4 for the meaning of these Sutra)

This is the state of ultimate spiritual absorption or Raja yoga. This is the state when the meditator becomes one with the object. It is a transcendental stage that is to be **experienced**. To convey that experience in words is not possible.

But still, let's try to understand this experience by the example of candle meditation or Jyoti Trataka.

When we sit in front of the candle and focus on it, the first thing which will disturb us is the outside objects, such as noise, insects, heat /cold, etc. so we try to fully concentrate on the object and not get affected by the sense. This is the practice of Pratyahara / Withdrawal of senses.

Now let's say we master the pratyahara, the sense objects do not disturb us anymore, and when we sit for the meditation, we can concentrate on the flame but there are still impressions of the outside world in the mind so even when we are trying to concentrate, there are various other thoughts keep coming in the mind. This is the stage of Dharana / Concentration.

Let's say we have mastered Dharana and now we can actually focus only on the flame. All the thoughts in the mind are now related to the flame. This is the stage of Dhyana / Meditation.

Then comes a stage, wherein we start feeling the heat of the candle within ourselves. As if we are the flame. This is the stage of being one with the object referred to as Samadhi.

Patanjali divides samadhi into 2 categories- **Sampragyata and Asampragyata.**

Sampragyata Samadhi refers to conscious meditation and Asampragyata Samadhi can be understood as a super-conscious meditation.

Sampragyata has 4 varieties/categories- **Vitarka, Vichara, Ananda, and Asmita.**

Vitarka-Vichar-Ananda-Asmita-Roopa-Anugamat-Sampragyata

||PYS 1.17||

Vitarka – Reasoning / analytical thinking, **Vichar** – Insight / Discrimation, **Ananda** - bliss, **Asmita** - I-ness / unqualified egoism, **Roop** - nature, **Anugamat** - accompanied by, **Sampragyata** – cognitive.

Meaning- Sampragyata samadhi is that which is accompanied by Vitarka, Vichara, Ananda, and Asmita.

Savitarka

- When the mind meditates upon an object again and again. By isolating it from other objects.
- When the mind thinks of elements of nature by thinking of their beginning and their end, this is one sort of Savitarka.

- **Questioning the elements**, as it were that they may give up their truths and their powers to the man who meditates upon them.

Savichar

When the meditation goes a step higher and takes the **Tanmatra as its object** and thinks of them as in time and space. It is called Savichar Samadhi.

Sanandam

The blissful samadhi or Sanandam is the next stage when the elements are given up and the object of meditation is the **thinking organ.**

Asmita

In this stage, **Satvik mind** is the object of meditation. In this stage, the sadhak can think of him/herself without the gross body. **Sadhaka now identifies him/herself with the sukshma sharira.**

Savitarka is gross Samadhi. Savichar is a subtle Samadhi. Sananda is deep subtle Samadhi. Asmita is still a deeper subtle Samadhi. These are all stages like the steps of an ascending staircase. All of these are also referred to as **Sabija Samadhi or Savikalpa Samadhi.**

Asampragyata

There is another Samadhi that is attained by the constant practice of cessation of all mental activity, in which the Chitta retains only the unmanifested impressions. This is called Asampragyata

Samadhi. This is also referred to as Nirbeeja Samadhi or Nirvikalpa Samadhi.

With constant practice of intense meditation and frequent detachment, sadhaka reaches the stage of Asampragyata Samadhi, where the mind becomes quiet and does not get any thoughts. Once Sadhaka comes back from the samadhi he/she remembers the stage of complete withdrawal from sense objects, with no thoughts but with a feeling. This feeling or experience is only felt because of the memory of it. Thus, in the state of Samadhi, the impression of complete emptiness is left. Therefore, after preventing all kinds of thoughts the state of empty mind samskaras is called Asampragyata Samadhi.

Dharma-Megha samadhi / Kaivalya

Prasankhyane-apy-akusidasy-sarvatha-vivekakh-yater-dharmameghah-samadhih ||PYS 4.29||

Meaning- Even when arriving at the right discriminating knowledge of the senses, he who gives up the fruits, unto him comes as the result of perfect discrimination, the Samadhi called the **Dharm-Megha-Samadhi.**

This stage is considered the highest enlightened state of human existence. All the previously explained Samadhi states have some associated fruits, referred to as **Vibhuti.** These Vibhutis depend upon the object of meditation as explained in the Vibhuti Pada.

When Sadhaka attains a particular samadhi Avastha, he/she receives the Vibhuti. At this time, if the sadhak chooses to ignore the Vibhuti and stays on the path of liberation only then can he/she move on to the next stage. Indulging in the Vibhuti is highly discouraged on the path of Moksha, especially when it is done for public attention.

Dharma Megha Samadhi is the highest stage when the sadhaka has crossed all the stages without getting distracted by any Vibhuti on the path.

Concept of mental well-being according to Patanjali Yoga.

- Patanjali emphasizes following **Abhyasa** (relentless positive self- effort) and **vairagya** (dispassionate attitude).
- Along with abhyasa and vairagya, one should also follow **Ishwara Pranidhana** to become mentally balanced.
- He provides an antidote to the stress by suggesting a change in our inner perspective through **Pratipaksha Bhavanam** (adopting contrary attitudes in the face of negativities).
- He advises us to develop clarity of mind through **Chitta Prasadanam**.
- Through the practice of **Ashtanga Yoga** all the aspects of human wellbeing can be taken care of.

2.6 Hatha Yoga: Parampara and Basic Yoga Texts

Origin

- The earlier eras (Before the Post-Classical Period) saw yogis laying emphasis only on **meditation and contemplation**. Yogic practices were more like moral codes. Mental practices were emphasized. But during the Post-Classical period, yogis began to probe the hidden powers of the body and **Tantra Yoga** was developed. Tantra Yoga was then foreseen to be

misunderstood by the people and the mystic practices were removed from it, and what **remained is called Hatha Yoga.**
- Hatha Yoga is said to be propounded by Lord Shiva himself as Adi yogi.
- The Nath Yogis of the Hatha Yoga tradition such as **Matsyendranath** was given the utmost respect. He is considered 2nd after Shiva (Adi yogi). **Gorakshanath** was his prime disciple.
- Matsyendranath is also known as Minanath
- The oldest dated text so far found to describe Hatha Yoga is the 11th-century Amrit Siddhi, but it is believed that the teachings and practices of Hatha Yoga are even older than that.
- Various Hatha yoga texts mentioned that the **prime aim** of Hatha yoga is **to achieve Raja yoga.**
- According to the prominent **Sage Yajnavalkya**, Hatha Yoga should be taught only to that person, who follows the practices mentioned in the holy scripture (the Vedas), who is desireless, who observes Yamas and Niyama, who keeps away from bondage, who conquers the anger, who dedicated him/her self at the feet of his /her guru, etc.

Modern Developments

- In 1918 The Yoga Institute was officially founded in Mumbai by Shri Yogendra.
- In the 1920s the renowned Krishnamacharya started Hatha Yoga School in Mysore. However, his students were taught in the Mysore style, which is non-standardized. Krishnamacharya taught such famous devotees as **Indra Devi, T.K.V. Desikachar, Sri K. Pattabhi Jois, and B.K.S. Iyengar** who all created their

own styles of teachings and spread the practice throughout the world.
- In 1924, **Kaivalyadham Yoga Research Institute** was established by Swami Kuvalyananda.
- In 1936, Swami Sivananda founded **Divine Life Society.**

Meaning of Hatha Yoga

The word Hatha means wilful or forceful and hence Hatha Yoga is sometimes understood as Yoga that involves tremendous willpower and determination. But the more appropriate meaning of hatha yoga comes from the two Bija mantras- **"Ha" and "Tha"**

- **"Ha"**- Solar energy- Pingala nadi- Masculine Aspect- Right nostril
- **"Tha"**- Lunar energy- Ida nadi- Feminine Aspect- Left nostril

Through Hatha, a **balance** between Ida and Pingala can be achieved which then activates a very significant Nadi called **Sushumna**. It's the opening of this Nadi (Sushumna), which raises the possibilities of higher human functioning.

hakara- kirtitah- suryah- thakarsh- chandra- uchyate |

surya- chandra- masoryogat- hatha- yogo- nigadyate ||

Meaning- "Ha" kara is the sound of Surya (sun) and "Tha" kara is the sound of Chandra (moon). The aim of Hatha Yoga is to balance these energies so that prana can flow through Sushumna.

Ashtama Siddhis

Various Hatha yoga texts such as Hatha Pradipika say one can achieve **Ashtama Siddhis** if one is adept in Hatha yoga. These are-

- **Anima** - To be able to become as small as an atom
- **Laghima**- To be able to become weightless
- **Mahima**- To be able to become as large as the universe
- **Garima**- To be able to become the heaviest
- **Prapti**- To be able to reach any place
- **Prakamya**- To be able to stay underwater and maintain the body and youth
- **Vashitva**- Control over all objects, organic and inorganic
- **Ishatva**- To be able to create and destroy at will.

Structure of a hatha abhyas

- The Hatha school offers a wide understanding of human anatomy. It offers ways to clean the internal organs **(Shat Kriyas)**.
- It also suggests physical postures **(Asana)** to strengthen the muscles and joints.
- Then it moves to even subtler systems of Nadi and offers ways to cleanse and balance the Nadi **(Pranayama)**.
- Then it gives ways to control and channel the energy/prana shakti at designated places in the body **(Mudras & Bandhas)**.
- Once all this is mastered one can move to the deeper practice of gathering within and listening to oneself **(Meditation)**.
- So, to put together, Hatha yoga usually consists of
  - **Shat Kriyas - Purification (Shodhana)**
  - **Asana - Strength & Disease-free (Dhridhta)**

- Pranayama- Lightness (Laghatvam)
- Mudras & Bandhas - Steadiness (Sthairyam)
- Meditation - Liberation (Nirliptam)

Different teachers of Hatha yoga have suggested their own perspectives on the practice but the basic structure of practice remains the same. For instance-

- A very prominent teacher of Hatha yoga, **Sage Swatmaram Suri (author of Hatha Yoga Pradipika)** says that one should only do Shat Kriyas if there is any illness in the body. Otherwise one can directly begin with Asanas. So, the structure suggested by him has 4 steps and is popularly known as **Chaturanga Yoga-**
    - **Asana (15)** - To achieve strength & disease-free state of body
    - **Pranayama (8)**- To achieve lightness in the body
    - **Mudra & Bandha (10)** - To achieve Steadiness in the body
    - **Nadanusandhana** -To achieve liberation

- Another prominent teacher, **Sage Gheranda (author of Gheranda Samhita),** made Shat Kriyas a mandatory practice and also added more practices to internalize oneself, as a preparatory for Samadhi. The structure suggested by him has 7 steps and is known as **Saptanga Yoga or Ghatasya Yoga.**
    - **Shat Kriyas (6)** - To achieve **Purification / Shodhanam** of the body.
    - **Asana (32)** - To achieve **Strength / Dhridhta** in the body.
    - **Mudra (25)** - To achieve **Steadiness / Sthairyam** in the body.
    - **Pratyahara** - To achieve **Calming / Dhairyam** in the body.

- **Pranayama (8)**- To achieve **Lightness / Laghatvam** in the body.
- **Dhyana (3)** - To achieve **Realization of the self / Pratyaksham**.
- **Samadhi (6)**- To achieve the **Isolation / Nirliptam**

2.7 Hatha Yoga, Ref: Hatha Yoga Pradipika (HYP)

Hatha Yoga Pradipika is a text written by **Swami Swatmaram** somewhere in the 15th century. The text is a very reliable source of information on traditional Hatha yoga sadhana. This is comprised of 4 chapters and the structure of practice is referred as **Chaturanga Yoga.**

Chapter 1- Asana, **Chapter 2-** Shatkarma and Pranayama, **Chapter 3-**Mudra and Bandha, **and Chapter 4-** Samadhi

Swatmaram clarifies at the beginning of the book that the aim of Hatha yoga is to achieve Raja Yoga.

Chapter 1- Asana

Asana practice brings Dridhta (strength) to the body. HYP mentions 15 asanas.

Swastikasana (The auspicious pose)-

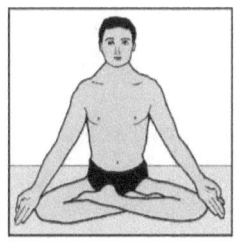

Technique-

Placing both the soles of the feet on the inner side of the thighs, sitting equipoised with a straight body. This is called Swastikasana.

Benefits- The sciatic nerve is gently massaged, thereby influencing the whole lumbar region. The abdominal muscles are also influenced and the inner body temperature is affected.

The symbol of the swastika represents **fertility, creativity, and auspiciousness**, thus this asana, being so named induces the same capacity in the body.

Gomukhasana (Cow's face pose)

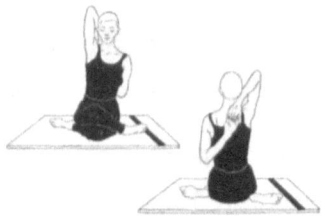

Technique- Placing the right ankle next to the left buttock and the left ankle next to the right buttock is called Gomukhasana.

Benefits- This tones the muscles and nerves around the shoulders and cardiac plexus, reproductive organs and glands.

On the pranic level, Gomukhasana affects the **Vajra nadi** and prevents prana from flowing outward. Instead, prana is directed to and accumulated in Mooladhar Chakra.

Because the **fingers are interlinked**, Prana also cannot escape through the hands. this asana creates a **complete energy circuit.**

Veerasana (hero's pose)

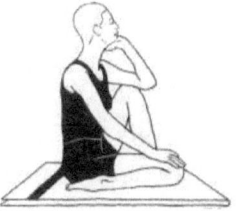

Technique- Placing one foot by the opposite thigh and the other foot under the same thigh is Veerasana.

Placing the left foot below the left buttocks and the right foot over the left thigh and keeping the knees widely spread **is another variation.**

This is also known as **Mahaveerasana.**

Benefits- Veerasana stabilizes the energy flow to the reproductive organs and enables control of sexual energy.

It increases **willpower** and strengthens the body.

Koormasana (tortoise pose)

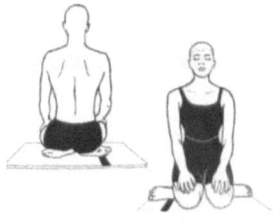

Technique- Press the anus firmly with the ankles positioned in opposite directions and sit well poised.

In another variation, Sit on the buttocks with legs spread in front of you, slip the arms under the knees, take the hands back behind the buttocks, and interlock the fingers.

Benefits- Very effective posture to correct the curved spine. People suffering from a lack of energy, and sexual and urinary disorders can practice this asana to rectify these problems.

Kukkutasana (cockerel pose)

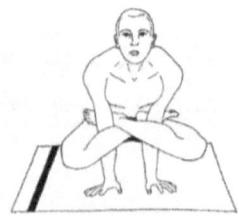

Technique- Assuming padmasana insert the hands between the thighs and calves, planting the palms firmly on the ground, raise the body in the air.

Benefits- This asana is said to be useful in the process of awakening Kundalini. It strengthens the arms and shoulder muscles and gives the sensation of levitation.

Uttankoormasana (Stretching tortoise pose)

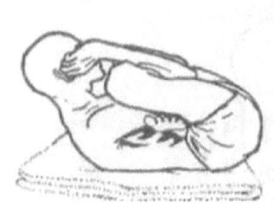

Technique- Sitting in Kukkutasana, place both hands at the shoulders/ears and lie flat on the back like a Tortoise.

In another variation, Lie down bring the knees to the chest and perform Padmasana and perform Kukkutasana now and hold the shoulders/ears. This is also called Garbhasana, the embryo poses.

Benefits- This asana tones the nervous system and induces relaxation if the final position is held comfortably.

Dhanurasana (Bow pose)

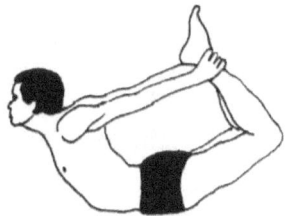

Technique- Lying down in a prone position, bend your knees and hold your toes with both palms and draw them to your ears. In this asana, one should concentrate on Vishuddhi Chakra, Manipur Chakra, or on the midpoint where the back is bending.

Benefis

- Very effective in the management of diabetes as it massages the liver and pancreas.
- The whole alimentary canal is toned along with kidney stimulation.
- Helpful in correcting hunched back and dropping shoulders.
- Helps in correcting menstrual issues and female infertility
- Stimulates solar plexus.

- Stimulates and regulates the endocrine gland, particularly the Thyroid Gland and Adrenal Gland and it induces the production of Cortisone.

Matsyendrasana (Spinal twist pose)

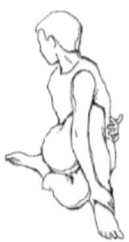

Technique- Sit with the legs straightened in front of you. Bend your right leg and place the right foot across the left thigh. Fold your left leg placing the left foot beside the right hip. Twisting the torso place the right arm behind the body and grab the right heel with the left palm crossing the right knee with the left elbow.

Benefits-

- Increase digestive fire.
- Helps in awakening dormant energy centers.
- Brings equilibrium to the Bindu and prevents it from mixing with the gastric fire.
- It stimulates the Pancreas, Liver, Spleen, Kidney, Stomach, and Ascending, and Descending colons.
- Useful in the treatment of diabetes, Constipation, Dyspepsia, and urinary problems along with lumbago, rheumatism, and slipped disc.

Paschimottanasana (Back stretching pose)

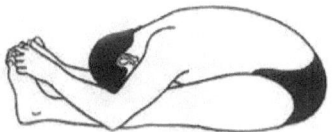

Technique- Stretching the legs on the ground like a stick, bending forward, holding the toes with both hands, and placing the forehead on the knees is called Paschimottasana.

Benefits

- This posture stretches the whole spinal column and central nervous system through which Sushumna runs thus enabling nervous and pranic impulses to pass directly up to the higher centers.
- Very effective in the yogic management of digestive disorders, diabetes, constipation, flatulence, and loss of appetite, as it manages and stimulates all the organs inside the stomach. Also helpful in regulating the menstrual cycle.

Mayurasana (Peacock Pose)

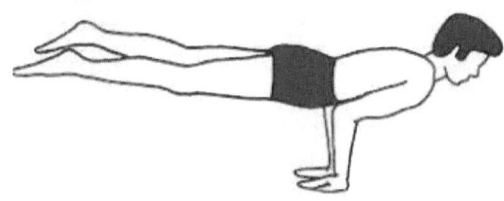

Technique- Lie on the stomach, placing both hands on the ground (under the body) and the elbows at the sides of the navel. Raise the body high, keeping it like a stick. This is called the Mayurasana by the exponents of yoga.

Benefits

- Helps in treatment of the enlargement of the gland.
- Rectifies the imbalance of vata, pitta, and Kapha.
- The digestion becomes so strong that it can even digest the **deadliest poison (Kalkuta).**
- Helps in constipation, flatulence, indigestion, dyspepsia, chronic gastritis, and diabetes.

Shavasana (Corpse Pose)

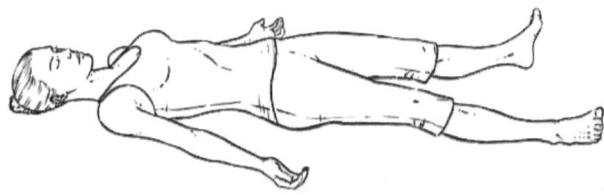

Technique- Lying flat on the ground with the face upward, in the manner of a dead body, is called Shavasana.

Benefits- It removes fatigue and gives rest to the mind. Very effective for developing Dharana and Dhyana.

Siddhasana (The adept pose)

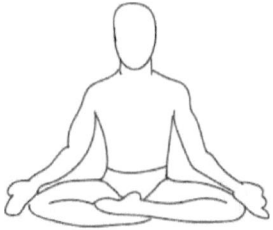

Technique- Press the perineum with the heel of one foot. Place the other foot on the top of the genitals. Having done this, rest the chin on the chest. Remaining still and steady with the senses controlled, gaze steadily into the eyebrow center, it breaks open the door to liberation.

For women, Siddha yoni asana is suggested. The lower heel is pressed into the opening of the vagina and the upper heel rests against the clitoris. The toes of both feet are inserted between the thighs and calf muscles.

Benefits

- It purifies 72000 nadis.
- 12 years + Right Food + Contemplation on self = success in yog.
- If one can master this asana one will acquire siddhis.
- On a pranic level, Siddhasana balances the alternating flow of Ida and Pingala nadis, thus activating Sushumna.
- Swatmaram says that Siddhasana is also known as Vajrasana, Muktasana, or Guptasana. (These are explained as separate asanas in Gherand Samhita)

- **Out of these 15 asanas, Swatmaram considers Siddhasana to be the most important asana.**
- It is said that there is no asana like Siddhasana, no kumbhak like Kevala, no mudra like Khechri, and no Laya like Nada (Anahata nada).

Padmasana (Lotus Pose)

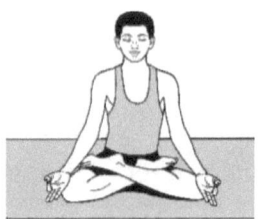

Technique- Place the right foot on the left thigh and the left foot on the right thigh, cross the hands behind the back, and firmly hold the toes. Press the chin against the chest and look at the tip of the nose. This is called padmasana, the destroyer of a yogi's disease.

Benefits

- This is called the destroyer of disease.
- This asana changes the metabolic structure and brain patterns and helps create balance in the whole system.
- This is also helpful for people with emotional and nervous disorders. However, people with sciatica or sacral infection should not do Padmasana until the problems is alleviated.

Simhasana (Lion's pose)

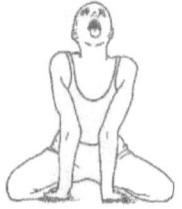

Technique

Place the ankles below the scrotum. Right ankle on the left side, left ankle on the right side of the perineum. Place the palms on the knees, fingers spread apart, keep the mouth open and gaze at the nose tip with a concentrated mind.

In another technique place the right foot under the right hip and the left under the left, and separate the knees widely. This is the sitting position of Bhadrasana. Place the palms on the knees or on the floor. Keeping the elbows straight and raising the chin 2/3 inches, practice Shambhavi Mudra, and extend the tongue as far as is comfortable. Inhale deeply through the nose and exhale making a roaring sound like a lion.

This technique is helpful in toning the throat and eradicating stammering. This is more effective in front of the rising sun.

Benefits- Useful for alleviating numerous throat, mouth, nose, and ear diseases. It helps to **externalize introverted people.**

Bhadrasana (Gracious pose)

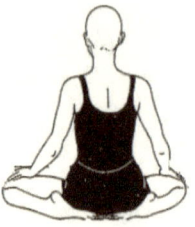

Technique- Place the ankles below the genitals on the sides by the perineum, the left ankle on the left side, right by the right. Then hold the feet and remain motionless.

This is also called **Gorakshasana**. Some call it **Mulabandhasana.**

Benefits- It tones reproductive organs. Other benefits are similar to Padmasana, Siddhasana, and Vajrasana.

This chapter also explains the Sadhak tattva (Cause of success) and Badhak tattva (Cause of failure), Yama (Social observances), Niyama (Personal Observances), Matha (Living situation of a Hatha Yogi), Pathya & Apathya Bhojan (Prescribed & Prohibited Food), Mitahara (Moderate Food), etc.

Yama And Niyama

There are some fundamental principles that a Hatha yogi should follow, these are referred to as Yama and Niyama-

Yama (10)- Rules of social conduct

Ahimsa-Satyam-Asteyam-Brahmcharyam-Kshama-Dhritih |

Daya-ārjavam-Mitahara-Śhaucham-Chaivam-Yama-Dashah ||

Meaning- (In the same order as shloka)- Non-violence, Truth, Non-stealing, Continence (being absorbed in a pure state of consciousness), Forgiveness, Endurance, Compassion, Humility / Honesty, Humbleness, Moderate Diet, and Cleanliness are the ten rules of social conduct.

Niyama (10)- Rules of personal conduct

Tapah-Santosh-Astikyam-Danam-Ishwarpujanam Sidhant Vakya Shravanam- Hri- Mati cha-japo-Hutam Niyama Dashah- Samprokta- Yogshashtra- Vishardaih ||

Meaning- (In the same order as shloka)- Austerity, contentment, faith in the supreme God, charity, worship of God, listening to the recitations of sacred scriptures, modesty, a discerning intellect, mantra repetition, and sacrifice (yajna) are the 10 personal observances.

Sadhaka and Badhaka Tattva

Sadhaka Tattva- (Facilitating elements in the path of Yoga)

Utsahat-Sahasa-Dhairya-TattvaJnanasch-Nishchyat ||

Jana sangha-Parityaga-Shadbhiryogah-Prasidhyati ||HYP 1.16||

Meaning- (In the same order as shloka)- Enthusiasm, Courage, Perseverance, Discrimination, Determination, and Avoiding the company of common people are the causes of success for the yogi.

Badhak Tattva- (Obstructing elements in the path of Yoga)

Atyaharah Prayasacha Prajalpo Niyamagraha |

Jansanghsch Lolyam cha Shadbhiryogah Vinashyati ||1.15||

Meaning- (In the same order as shloka)- Overeating, Over-exertion, Talkativeness, Over-adhering to the rules, The company of common people, and an Unstable attitude are the causes of failure for the yogi.

Note: Analyse the Yama, Niyama, and Sadhak-Badhak Tattva of Hatha with the Yama-Niyama, and Antarayas of Patanjali Yoga Sutra. It will help you remember these from both texts.

Concept of Matha (Living Situation)-

Sage Swatmaram gives specific guidelines in Hatha Yoga Pradipika for the living situation of the yogi –

- The Hatha yogi should live alone in a Hermitage / Matha.
- The length of the practice place should be a bow (one and a half meters), where there are no surrounding objects which may cause physical affliction.
- One should also practice in this same place every day,
- Yogi should live in a well-administered and virtuous kingdom (nation or town) where good alms can be easily attained.
- The room of the yogi should have a small door without an aperture (window), holes, or cracks.
- It should be neither too high nor too low.
- It should be spotlessly clean, wiped with cow manure, and free from animals or insects.
- Outside of the Matha, there should be an open platform with a thatched roof.
- There should be a well outside and it should be protected with a surrounding wall/fence.
- The appearance of the hermitage should be pleasant.

It is important to understand that these guidelines are in **the context of ancient times**. The idea was to live in a place where food and water are easily available and yogi has a secluded and safe atmosphere for the practice.

Mitahara- Swatmaram defines Mitahara as-

Susnigdham- Madhuram- Aharascha- Chaturthansha-Vivarjitah |

Bhujyate-Shiva-Samprityai-Mitaharah-Sa-Uchyate ||HYP 1.59||

Meaning- Mitahara is defined as an agreeable (nutritious, sweet, lubricating) sweet food, leaving one-fourth of the stomach empty, and eaten as an offering (prasad) to please shiva **(Mindful eating / Bhav- Purna Bhojan).**

Apathya Bhojan (Prohibited Food)

kaṭu-āmla-tīkṣhṇa-lavaṇ-oṣhṇa-harīta-śāka- sauvīra-taila-tila-sarṣhapa-madya-matsyān |

ājādi-māṃsa-dadhi-takra-kulattha-kola- piṇḍyāka- hingghu-laśunādyam - apathyamāhuḥ || HYP 1.61 ||

Meaning- (As per the order in the shloka) Bitter, sour, Pungent, saltish, hot, green vegetables (apart from the ones which are prescribed), fermented, oily, mixed with sesame seed, Mustard seed, intoxicating liquors, fish, the meat of goat, etc. curd, Butter-milk, horse gram (Dolichos Uniflorus), juju berry (A type of plum), oil-cake, asafœtida (hînga), garlic, onion, etc., should not be eaten.

> Swatmaram says that food which is reheated, which is dry (devoid of natural oil), which is excessively salty or acidic, stale, or has too many mixed vegetables is considered unhealthy for a hatha yogi.

Pathya Food (Prescribed food)

ghodhūma-śhāli-yava-ṣhāṣhṭika-śobhanā-annaṃ kṣhīr-ājya-khaṇḍa-navanīta-sita-madhūni |

śuṇṭhī-paṭolakaphalādika-pañcha-śākaṃ- mudghādi-divyamudakaṃ cha yamīndra-pathyam || HYP 1.65 ||

Meaning- (As per the order in the shloka) The most conducive food for yoga are- grains like wheat (godhum), Rice (Shali), and Barley (Yava), all of them belonging to the category of grains that ripen in 60 days. Milk (kshir), clarified butter (ghee), Crystallized sugar (Ajya), Butter (Navneet), White Sugar (Sita), Honey (Madhuni), Dry Ginger (Shunthi), panch shak, Mung (Mudga), Divyam Udkam (Rainwater).

> **Panch shak- (Five prescribed vegetables for a hatha yogi)**
>
> 1. Patolak fal - parval, 2. Kalsak- a variety of jute, 3. Vastak - bathua, 4. Himlochika- a medicinal plant also used as a food source, 5. Balsak- another medicinal plant)
>
> The name of the panch shaka is given in **Gherand Samhita**
>
> Swatmaram says that The yogi should take nourishing and sweet food mixed with ghee and milk, it should nourish the Dhatus and should be pleasing and suitable.

Chapter 2- Shatkarma And Pranayama

Note: The detailed information on Shatkarma in comparison with Gherand Samhita is mentioned in Unit 1.10

Pranayama

- Hatha Yoga Pradipika refers to Pranayama as **Kumbhaka**. Swatmaram emphasizes the retention of breath in the combination of the bandhas.
- However, for general practice, in the beginning, it is advised to practice these without retention and without bandha. One should slowly build up the capacity of retaining the breath in and then the bandhas practice can be done.
- Swatmaram says that Retention should be practiced perfectly four times a day: Early morning (Before Sunrise), midday, evening and midnight. The aim is to achieve eighty counts of retention.
- There are **8 types** of Kumbhaka- **Surya Bheda, Ujjayi, Seetkari, Sheetali, Bhastrika, Bhramri, Moorchha, Plavini**

SuryaBheda- (Vitality Stimulating pranayama)

- Sit in any meditative asana. Keep the left palm in Dhyana Mudra and the right palm in Nasikagra or Pranava Mudra.
- Now, close the left nostril with the ring finger and inhale through the right nostril.
- Apply Jalandhar Bandha and then moola bandha and hold your breath up to capacity.
- Then, first release the Moola Bandha, then the Jalandhar Bandha, and exhale through the left nostril.

Note- SuryaBheda can **also be practiced** by inhaling and exhaling through the right nostril only. However, when you breathe only through the right nostril, this might **shut off Ida Nadi** and the functions of the left nostril. By exhaling through the left nostril, you release energy and any impurities that remain in Ida. By inhaling through the right nostril, you draw the prana into Pingala, and by retaining the breath after inhalation, you keep the prana in Pingala.

Benefits

- Surya Bheda is excellent for purifying the cranium.
- Destroying imbalances of the wind doshas and eliminating worms of intestines.
- This pranayama helps in making introverted people extroverts.
- Prevents old age and death, and increases body heat.

Contraindication

- This is contraindicated for people with epilepsy, heart disease, anxiety, and high blood pressure.
- One should avoid practicing it late at night as it may make it more difficult to fall asleep.

Chandra-Bhedi Pranayama- If the Suryabhedi pranayama is practiced in a reverse manner, inhaling through the left nostril and exhaling through the right, it activates Ida Nadi and is known as Chandrabhedi pranayama. In the HYP as well as in Gheranda Samhita, nothing has been written about this pranayama because if Ida is awakened the mind can introvert completely and the body will become lethargic. It is quite safe to activate Pingala Nadi through SuryaBheda pranayama, but it can be dangerous to activate Ida through Chandrabheda unless the guru has specifically advised it

Ujjayi- (Psychic Breathing / Ocean breath)

- Sit in any meditative asana. Keep the left palm in Dhyana Mudra and the right palm in Nasikagra or Pranava Mudra. Keep the palms on the knees.
- Now, close the mouth and breath through both nostrils, gently contracting the glottis and making a snoring sound from the back of the throat.
- Apply Jalandhar Bandha and then moola bandha and hold your breath up to capacity.
- Then, first release the Moola Bandha, then the Jalandhar Bandha, and exhale through the left nostril.

Benefits

- This is an excellent pranayama to stimulate the Thyroid gland.
- This removes phlegm from the throat and stimulates the digestive fire.

- It is highly recommended for people suffering from insomnia and mental tension.
- It removes dropsy and disorders of the Nadis and Dhatu.
- This pranayama can be done while moving, standing, sitting, or walking.

Contraindication

- Anyone with low blood pressure should first correct the condition and then attempt the practice.
- Anyone with heart disease should not combine bandha and breath retention in this Pranayama.

Seetkari (The hissing breath)

- Sit in any meditative asana. Keep both palms in dhyana mudra.
- This pranayama is done through the mouth. Open the lips wide but keep the teeth clenched.
- Draw the breath in through the mouth making a hissing sound,
- Apply Jalandhar Bandha and then moola bandha and hold your breath up to capacity.
- Then, first release the Moola Bandha, then the Jalandhar Bandha, and exhale through both nostrils.

Benefits

- This pranayama has a cooling effect on the body and hence is effective in controlling fever. It also brings control over hunger, thirst, sleep, and laziness.
- This establishes harmony in the endocrine system and regulates the hormonal secretions of the reproductive organs.

- Helps in curing enlarged gland issues such as an enlarged stomach, enlarged spleen, etc.

Contraindication

- Do not practice in cold weather, low blood pressure, cold, or sneezing.
- Since this is mouth breathing, the air doesn't get cleaned (as it does when breathing through the nose) hence do not practice in a dirty, polluted atmosphere.
- Do not practice in case of chronic constipation because this pranayama reduces the heat produced in the lower energy centers, particularly those connected to the reproductive and excretory organs.

Sheetali (The cooling breath)

- Sit in any meditative asana. Keep both palms in dhyana mudra.
- This one is also done through the mouth. Taking the tongue out, roll it as if you are trying to whistle (Kaki mudra).
- Inhale through the tongue and retain the breath.
- Apply Jalandhar Bandha and then moola bandha and hold your breath up to capacity.
- Then, first release the Moola Bandha, then the Jalandhar Bandha, and exhale through both nostrils.

Benefits & Contraindication- Same as Seetkari.

Note: Seetkari and Sheetali are basically the same pranayama techniques with slight differences. in Seetkari the awareness is focused on the hissing sound and in the Sheetali it is kept on the cooling sensation of the breath.

Bhastrika (Bellows Breath)

- Sit in any meditative asana preferably padmasana. Keep both palms in dhyana mudra.
- Inhale and exhale the air through the nostrils repeatedly like a pair of bellows being pumped.
- Once the intended counts are completed or when the body is tired, inhale through the right nostril using Nasikagra mudra, hold the breath up to capacity, apply Jalandhar Bandha, and then moola bandha.
- Then, first release the Moola Bandha, then the Jalandhar Bandha, and exhale through the left nostril.
- This pranayama increases the heat in the body; hence it should be followed by a few rounds of Sheetali / Seetkari pranayama, especially in the warm season.

Benefits

- This pranayama heats the nasal passages and sinuses, clearing away excess mucus and building up resistance to colds and all respiratory disorders.
- Improves digestion and stimulates a sluggish system.
- It increases the appetite, accelerates the metabolic rate, and strengthens the nervous system.

Contraindication

People with high blood pressure, heart disease, brain tumor, vertigo, stomach or intestinal ulcers, glaucoma, dysentery, or diarrhea must not attempt this practice.

Bhramari- This pranayama is done usually assuming the Shanmukhi mudra (closing the five senses with five fingers), some also do this by just closing the ears with the index finger.

- Sit in any meditative asana.
- Place your thumb on the ears, index fingers on the forehead, middle fingers on the eyes, ring fingers by the sides of the nostrils, and little fingers by the side of the mouth (**Shanmukhi mudra**).
- Close your ear consciously with the thumbs in a way that you cannot hear any outside sound. Now inhale making a reverberating sound like the male bee and exhale slowly while softly making the sound of a female bee.
- This pranayama is also done with the Om chanting.

Benefits- This pranayama induces pratyahara. It helps to awaken the psychic sensitivity and awareness of subtle vibrations. The sound produced in Bhramari is very soothing and thus the practice relieves mental tension, and anxiety and reduces anger.

Contraindications- None.

Moorchha (Swooning Breath)- This is an **advanced pranayama**, the practice of which is to be done only under the supervision of a realized teacher

- Sit in any meditative asana. Keep both palms in dhyana mudra.
- Inhale and assume Jalandhar bandha then hold your breath until you start getting the faint feeling, as the name suggests moorchha, meaning to faint or to swoon. This is Moorchha Pranayama.

- Then release the Jalandhar bandha, raise the chin slightly, and exhale in a very controlled manner.
- The sensation of fainting occurs for two reasons. One is that continued retention lowers the oxygen concentration in the blood reaching the brain, i.e., hypoxia. Second, by compressing the vessels in the neck, Jalandhar bandha influences the pressure receptors in neck walls and the heart rate and the blood pressure are adjusted by the reflex response.

Benefits

- This pranayama prepares the mind for meditation.
- It helps reduce anxiety and mental tension.
- It induces relaxation and inner awareness.

Contraindication- Anyone suffering from heart disease, high blood pressure, or vertigo should not attempt this practice.

Plavini (Gulping Breath)- This is another **advanced pranayama**, which is rarely taught, and very little has been written about it. The practice of which is to be done only under the supervision of a realized teacher.

- Inhale the air by making kaki mudra and gulp it down the stomach.
- Repeat this until the stomach is all filled with air and hold until capacity and then exhale through both nostrils.

Benefits

- Plavana means to float. Success in this pranayama enables one to float on water.
- This is useful in cases of gastritis and stomach acidity.

- Traditionally, some yogis practice Plavini before going into samadhi for days together so that the stomach remains full during their natural fast.

Chapter 3- Mudra And Bandha

Mudra- Mudra means "gesture" or "attitude". A mudra may involve the whole body in a combination of asana, pranayama, bandha, and visualization techniques, or it may be a simple hand position. In the mudra, we let the prana flow in the chosen area of the body.

Bandha- Bandha means "to lock" or "to tighten". The bandhas aim to lock the pranas in particular areas and redirect their flow into Sushumna Nadi for spiritual awakening.

There are 10 mudras mentioned in Hatha Yoga Pradipika-

Mahamudra-Mahabandho-Mavedhascha-Khechari |

Uddiyanam-Moolabandhascha-Bandho-Jalandhar-bhidhah ||HYP 3.6||

Karani Vipareetakhyam Vajroli Shaktichalanam |

Idam hi Mudra-Dashakam-Jara-Maran-Nashakam ||HYP 3.7||

Mahamudra (The Great Attitude)

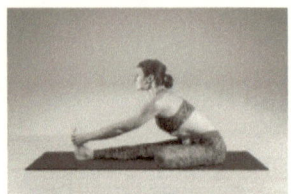

Practice-

- Sit with both legs stretched. Bend the left knee placing the left heel firmly into the perineum (At the location of the Mooladhar Chakra). keep the right leg straight on the ground.
- Inhale and perform Khechari mudra. Exhale and bend forward clasping the right toe with both hands.
- Keep the head erect and back straight. Slowly inhale and tilt the head slightly back. Perform Shambhavi mudra and then moola bandha.
- Hold your breath in and rotate the awareness from the Ajna to Vishudhhi to Mooladhar, spending 1-2 seconds at every chakra.
- Release the Shambhavi mudra and then Moola bandha then slowly exhale and return to the upright position and release the Khechari mudra
- Repeat with the other leg and then with both legs stretched.

Benefits

- The disorders like Maha-klesha (Ignorance, ego, anger, hatred, and fear of death are 5 maha klesha) are destroyed. Increases awareness and induces spontaneous meditation.

- Death caused by old age is evaded.
- All kinds of food- bitter, sour, stale food and even poison get digested as if they were nectar.
- Diseases like skin disorders (Leprosy), constipation, glandular enlargement, indigestion, and many others get destroyed.

Contraindications - HBP, Eye surgeries such as cataract, or lens implant, Pregnancy, Mensuration.

Maha bandha (The Great Lock)

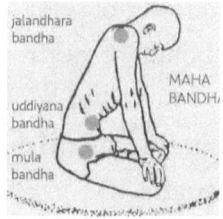

Practice-

- Place the left heel firmly at the region between the anus and penis (Perineum). Having placed the right foot on the left thigh.
- Then after inhalation performs Jalandhar bandha, moola bandha, and turn the mind into Shambhavi mudra. The air should be exhaled slowly after doing Kumbhak repeat with another side.
- As per Jyotsna (Commentary on HYP)- The Moolbandha happens by itself on the application of jiva bandha hence there is no need to apply Moolbandha once Jivhabandha is applied.

- Some guru says that there is no need for Jalandhar bandha. Applying Jivhabandha by pressing the tongue at the center of the Rajdanta (tooth) is comparatively simple.
- In Hatha Yoga Pradipika, Mahabandha is explained in 2 ways-
  - **With Antah Kumbhak**, applying Jalandhar Bandha, Mool Bandha, and Shambhavi Mudra.
  - **With Bahya Kumbhak,** applying Jalandhar, Uddiyana, and moola bandha.

Benefits

- Mahabandha is the bestower of great siddhis.
- This frees one from bonds of death and makes the 3 nadis unite in Ajna chakra.
- As per HYP Mahamudra and Mahabandha are unfruitful without Mahavedha mudra.

Maha Vedha (The Great Piercing Attitude)

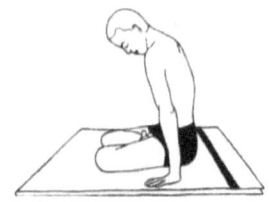

Practice-

Maintaining the Mahabandha place the palms by the sides of the thighs, keeping the elbows straight and slowly striking the ground with the buttocks. By doing so prana transcends the Ida and Pingala and enters into the central i.e., Sushumna nadi.

Benefits

- The practice of Mahavedha bestows great perfections.
- Mahamudra and Mahavedha are powerful techniques that introvert the mind and awaken psychic faculties. They affect the pineal and pituitary glands and thus the whole endocrinal system. Due to which hormonal secretions are regulated and catabolism is curtailed. Then the symptoms of old age such as wrinkles, grey hair, trembling etc. are either annihilated or reduced.
- **Mahabandha, Mahamudra, and Mahavedha are three great secrets that destroy old age and death, increase the digestive fire and bestow the Ashtama Siddhi.**
- These should be practiced daily at every yama (3-hour period i.e., 8 times a day).

Khechari (Attitude of dwelling in supreme consciousness)

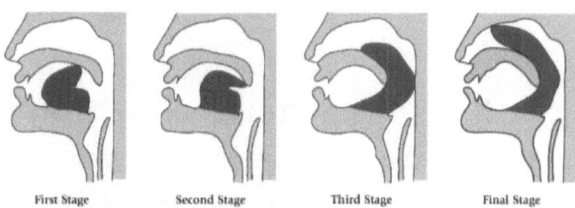

First Stage   Second Stage   Third Stage   Final Stage

Practice

- This is turning the tongue back into the cavity of the cranium and turning the eyes inwards towards the eyebrow center. This is also known as **Nabho mudra**.
- Swami Sivananda has called this practice **Lambhika Yog**.

- The other form of Khechari (Raja yoga form) is much simpler and can be performed by anyone. It is done by turning the tongue back so that the under surface touches the upper back portion of the soft palate and the tip of the tongue is inserted into the nasal orifice at the back of the throat if possible.

Benefits-

- The yogi who remains with the tongue going upwards for even half a second is freed from toxins, disease, death, old age, etc.
- When the upper cavity of the palate is sealed by Khechari mudra, the yogi develops immense Brahmcharya control.

Uddiyana Bandha

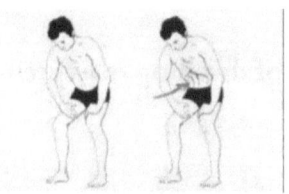

The word "Uddiyana" means "to rise up" or "to fly upward". This practice causes the diaphragm to rise towards the chest, hence the name. Uddiyana is often translated as the stomach lift. Another meaning is that the physical lock helps to direct prana into Sushumna Nadi so that it flows upward to the Sahasrara chakra. Uddiyana Bandha is practiced in Bahya Kumbhaka only. It stimulates the Manipura chakra.

Preparation- Uddiyana bandha must be practiced on an empty stomach. The bowels should be empty. **Agnisara Kriya** is an excellent preparatory practice.

Practice

- Stand tall with feet shoulder-width distance apart. Inhale through the nostrils and exhale bending forward from the waist, bringing the upper body parallel to the ground.
- Hold your breath out. Place the palms on the knees and keep the arms straight.
- Keeping the breath out, contract the abdomen muscles upwards and inwards towards the spine. Hold the lock for as long as possible, without straining.
- Slowly raise the body up, exhale slightly to release the lock on the lungs, and then slowly inhale through the nose.
- The same can be practiced sitting as well.

Benefits- The practice of this bandha destroys old age and helps one to conquer death. Stimulates digestive fire. Stimulates all the abdominal organs. Stimulates the solar plexus.

Contraindications- Colitis, Stomach or Intestinal ulcers, Hernia, HBP, Heart disease, Glaucoma, High intracranial pressure, Pregnancy.

Moola Bandha (Perineum / Cervix retraction lock)

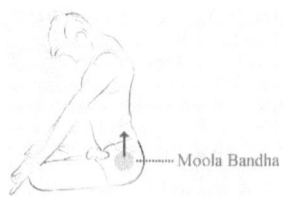
Moola Bandha

The word Moola means root / firmly fixed. Mooladhar refers to the root of the spine or the perineum where the seat of the kundalini or the primal energy is locked. Moola Bandha is effective in activating Mooladhar Chakra.

It is important to understand that moola bandha is a contraction of specific muscles in the pelvic floor, not the entire pelvic floor.

In the **male body**, the area of contraction is **between the anus and the testes.**

In the **female body**, the area of contraction is **behind the cervix**, where the uterus projects into the vagina.

With practice one becomes aware of these regions. **Ashwini and Vajroli** mudras can be performed as preparation for the Mooladhar bandha.

Practice

- Sit in a comfortable meditative asana, preferably Siddha / Siddha yoni asana.
- Close your eyes and bring awareness to the perineal. Inhale and hold your breath in, and contract the perineal/vaginal region by pulling up the muscles of the pelvic floor. Hold for as long as possible.
- Slowly release the bandha and exhale.
- Moola Bandha is usually practiced with Jalandhara Bandha in Antah kumbhak.
- Beginners can also practice rhythmic contraction and relaxation of pelvic floor muscles with normal breathing to build awareness and strength.

Benefits- Stimulates the pelvic nerves and tones the urogenital and excretory system. Induces sexual control. Destroys old age. Makes one grounded and stable.

Contraindication- Menstruation, Piles, HBP.

Jalandhar bandha (Throat Lock)

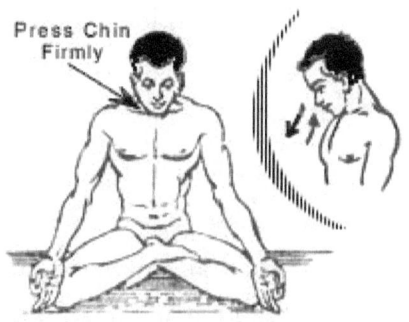

Contracting the throat by bringing the chin to the chest in Antar Kumbhaka / Bahya Kumbhaka, is called Jalandhar Bandha. This stimulates Vishuddhi Chakra. There are **2 interpretations** of its name-

1. Jalan means net and Dhara means stream or flow. The Jalandhara bandha is the lock that controls the network of Nadis in the neck. The physical manifestations of these Nadis are the blood vessels and nerves in the neck.
2. Alternatively- Jal means water. Jalandhara bandha is therefore the throat lock that holds the nectar or fluid flowing down to Vishuddhi from Bindu and prevents it from falling into the digestive fire. This is the way to boost the prana reservoir.

Practice

- Sit in any Siddhasana, Sidhayoni asana, Padmasana, Vajrasana or Sukhasana. Place the palm on the knees.
- Inhale and retain the breath and lower the chin against the chest in a way that you start feeling the pressure on the throat.
- Simultaneously, straighten and lock the elbows, press the knees down with the hands, and hunch the shoulders upwards and forward. Hold your breath for as long as you can.
- Then slowly bring the chin parallel to the ground, relax the shoulders, and exhale slowly through the nostrils

Benefits- The practice of this Bandha destroys all throat-related disorders. Removes old age and gives victory over death. Improves the functioning of the thyroid and parathyroid glands. Regular practice induces mental relaxation and relieves anxiety, stress, and hunger.

Contraindications- Cervical spondylosis, High intracranial pressure, Vertigo, Heart disease

Vipareeta Karani

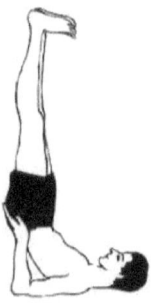

Practice

- When the navel region is above and the palate below, the sun is above and the moon below. It is called Vipreetkarni.

Benefits- This mudra destroys wrinkles and grey hair. Rejuvenates the body by getting rid of aging within **6 months of practice**. It balances the activities of the thyroid.

Contraindication- HBP, Heart disease, Glaucoma, Pregnancy, Mensuration.

Vajroli (Thunderbolt attitude)

Practice- By practicing gradual upwards contraction during the emission in intercourse, any man or woman achieves the perfection of Vajroli.

Benefits- By practicing this yogis can counter death.

Shakti Chalana (Attitude of moving the energy)

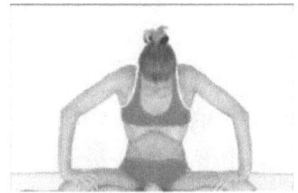

Practice

- Sit in Siddhasana.
- Inhale through the right nostril and perform Antar-kumbhak and Moolbandha.

- Exhale and perform Jalandhar and Uddiyana bandha.
- Then practice Nauli.
- Before inhaling, come back to Uddiyana, and slowly release Uddiyana and Jalandhar bandha.

Benefits- One who follows brahmacharya and always takes a moderate diet and practices arousal of kundalini achieves perfection in 40 days.

Imp- Various Names Of Kundalini- Kutilangi, Bhujangi, Shakti, Ishwari, Kundalini, Arundhati.

Chapter 4- Samadhi

In this chapter, **Nada-Anusandhana** is explained as it leads to samadhi. The word samadhi is made up of two roots- **Sama-** Equal and **Dhi-** Reflection or to perceive

There are **4 stages** of Nada-anusandhana:

Arambha - Avastha (Beginning Stage)- At this stage, the Brahma granthi gets pierced, and the feeling of bliss arises. Tinkling sounds and the unstruck sound (Anahata) are heard within the body.

Gatha- Avastha (Vessel Stage)- At this stage, Vishnu Granthi is pierced. From the Vishudhhi Chakra (Throat) the sound of the kettledrum manifests.

Parichaya - Avastha (Stage of Increase)- In this stage, one experiences the sound of the drum. This is the time of prana entering the Ajna Chakra, Imbalance of dosha, old age, disease, hunger, and sleep is overcome.

Nishpatti - Avastha (Stage of consummation)- At this stage, Rudra Granthi is pierced. The fire of Prana moves to the place of Ishwar. In this stage, Sadhak hears the sound of the flute and vina.

2.8 Hatha Yoga, Ref: Gheranda Samhita (GS)

Gherand Samhita is one of the classic texts of Hatha Yoga. It is in the form of a conversation between Sage Gheranda and his disciple Chandrakapali. Chandrakapali requested Sage Gheranda to give him the wisdom of yoga and Sage Gheranda explains to him this complete Yogic science.

At the beginning of the text, Sage establishes the importance of Yoga. He says

Nasti-Maya-samah-pasho nasti yogat-param-balam ||

Nasti- Jnanat-paro-bandhuh-na-ahamkarat-paro-ripuh ||GS 1.4||

Meaning- There are no shackles like Maya (illusion). There is no greater power than yoga, there is no greater friend than knowledge, and no enemy worse than egoism.

The text mentions a 7-limbed practice called **Saptanga Yoga** which is explained in 7 chapters. This structure is also referred to as **Ghatasya Yoga.**

Shatkarma- Shodhan (Purification), **Asana** - Dridhta (Strength), **Mudra** - Sthirta (Steadiness), **Pratyahara** - Dheerta (Calming), **Pranayama** - Laghatvam (Lightness), **Dhyan** - Pratyaksham (realization of the self), **Samadhi** - Nirliptam (Isolation)

Chapter 1- Shatkarma

Sage Gherand keeps Shatkarma as a **mandatory practice.** The 6 cleansing techniques are- Dhauti, Basti, Neti, Lauliki, Trataka, Kapalbhati.

Note: The detailed information on Shatkarma in comparison with HYP is mentioned in Unit 1, under topic 1.10

Chapter 2 -Asana

Sage Gherand says that there are as many asanas as species of animals. He gives the reference of Shiva Samhita saying that 84 lakhs asanas are mentioned by Shiva.

Out of them, 84 are regarded as important, and among these 84, he considered **32 asanas** are sufficient for practice. These are-

Siddham- Padhyam-Tatha-Bhadram-Muktam-Vajram-Cha-Swastikam|| Simham-Cha - Gomukham - Veeram - Dhanurasanam-Eva-Cha || GS 2.3||

Mritam - Guptam - Tatha - Matsyam - Matsyendrasanm- eve-cha|| Goraksham - Paschimottasnam - Utkatam - Sankatam – Tatha || GS 2.4||

Mayuram - Kukkutam - Kurmam - Tatha - Cha - Uttankurmakam ||

Uttan-Mandukam-Vriksham-Mandukam -Garunam-Vrisham ||GS 2.5||

Shalabham - Makaram - Cha - Ushtram - Bhujangam – Yogasanam || Dvatrishatam - Asanayeva - Martye - Siddhipradani - cha || GS 2.6||

Meaning- (In the same order as shloka)- Siddhasana, Padmasana, Bhadrasana, Muktasana, Vajrasana, Swastikasana, Simhasana, Gomukhasana, Veerasana, Dhanurasana, Mritasana (Shavasana), Guptasana, Matsyasana, Matsyendrasna, Gorakshasana, Paschimottasana, Utkatasana, Sankatasana, Mayurasana, Kukkutasana, Koormasana, Uttan-Koormasana, Uttanmadukasana, Vrikshasana, Mandukasana, Garudasana, Vrishasana, Shalabhasana, Makarasana, Ushtrasana, Bhujangasana, Yogasana are the 32 asana.

Chapter 3- Mudra & Bandha

The text mentions **25 mudra-**

Mahamudra - Nabhomudra - Uddiyanam - Jalandharam | Moolabandho - Mahabandho - Mahavedhascha - Khechari ||

Vipreetkarni - Yoni - Vajroli - Shaktichalni | Tadagi - Manduki Mudra - Shambhavi - Panchadharana ||

Ashvini - Pashini - Kaki - Matangi - Cha- Bhujangini | Panchavinshati - Mudras- cha - Siddhid - Iha - Yoginam ||

Meaning- (In the same order as shloka)- Mahamudra, Nabomudra, Uddiyana bandha, Jalandhar bandha, Moolabandha, Maha bandha, Mahavedha, Khechari, Vipreetkarni, Yoni mudra, Vajroli mudra, Shaktichalini, Tadagi mudra, Manduki mudra, Shambhavi mudra, Panchadharna (**Parthivi, Ambhasi, Vaishvnari, Vayavi, Nabho**), Ashwini mudra, Pashini mudra, Kaki mudra, Matangi mudra, Bhujangini mudra are the 25 mudras.

A comparative study of Mudra referencing from HYP and GS-

Name of the Mudra	Gheranda Samhita	Hatha Yoga Pradipika
Mahamudra (The Great Seal / Attitude)	Press the anus against the left heel and keep the right leg stretched. Grab the right toe with both hands, back straight, and gaze between the eye-brow (Bhru-Madhya Drishti).	The technique is the same as GS, but one of the commentaries on HYP suggest maintaining Moola bandha along with Khechari and Shambhavi Mudra.
Nabho-Mudra (Ether Seal)	Turn the tongue upwards and touch the roof of the mouth while retaining the breath.	Not Mentioned
Uddiyana Bandha (Flying-Up Lock)	This is done in Bahya Kumbhaka. It is the practice of drawing the stomach towards the spine.	Same Technique. HYP also mentions maintaining Jalandhar Bandha while holding this.

Jalandhar Bandha (Water- Pipe Lock)	Sitting in any Dhyana Asana, inhale and retain the breath. Then lower the chin to the chest, contracting the throat.	Same as GS
Moola Bandha (Root- Seal)	Press the perineum region against the left heel and right heel above the genitals. Contract the anus and press the navel against the spine.	The technique remains the same, HYP emphasizes on raising the **Apana** by contracting the rectum. Also, HYP says that Moola Bandha should be performed with Jalandhar Bandha during Antah-Kumbhaka and with Uddiyana Bandha and Jalandhar Bandha during Bahya Kumbhaka.

Mahabandha (The Great Lock)	Press the anus firmly by the left heel and press the right foot against the left heel. Contract the perineum and perform Jalandhar Bandha	Press the left heel against the perineum and place the right foot on the left thigh. Perform Antah Kumbhaka and adapt Jalandhar Bandha and Moola Bandh. Assume Shambhavi Mudra. HYP also says that there are some of the opinion about adapting the **Jivha Bandha (Keeping the tongue against the teeth)** instead of Jalandhar Bandha.

Maha Vedha (The Great Piercer)	Perform Maha Bandha and then add Uddiyana Bandha (Using Bahya Kumbhaka). **Sage Gheranda says that one who practices Maha Bandha, Moola Bandha, and Maha Vedha daily is the best yogi.**	Perform Maha Bandha and place the palms by the side of the body and gently tap the buttocks on the floor 3-7 times.
Khechari (Space-Walking Seal)	Slowly insert the tongue into the passage above the upper palate. Fix the gaze between the eyebrows.	Same as GS. **HYP also says that Khechari Mudra is also called Nabho Mudra and Swami Sivananda calls it Lambhika Yog.**
Vipreet-Karani (Inverse Action Seal)	Lie in supine position and raise the legs up and remain steady.	Same as GS

Yoni Mudra (**Perineal Seal**)	In Siddhasana, perform Shanmukhi mudra after inhaling through kaki mudra. Contemplate of Shiva-Shakti and on Shat- Chakras. The preliminary practice of Yoni mudra is **Shaktichalni.**	Not Mentioned
Vajroli (**Thunderbolt Attitude**)	Palms are on the floor and legs are crossed behind the neck and the body is lifted up pressing through the palms.	Slowly drawing in air through a prescribed tube inserted into the urethra of the penis. **HYP says that the perfection of Vajroli means being able to withdraw the seminal fluid during the height of climax. Vajroli for women is called Sahjoli.**

Shakti Chalana (Stirring the Power Seal)	Cover the midriff with a 9 inches long and 3 inches wide cloth and sit in Siddhasana. Inhale through both nostrils and forcibly join Prana and Apana. Then by Ashwini Mudra contract the anus till the Vayu is forced into the Sushumna. Then by restricting the Vayu, Kundalini feels choked ad rises upwards.	**Step 1-** Sit in Siddhasana and inhale through right nostril, perform Antah- Kumbhaka and Moola Bandha. Exhale and Perform Jalandhar and Uddiyana, then practice Nauli. Release Uddiyana and Jalandhar, raise the head and then inhale. **Step 2-** Sit in Vajrasana, grab the heels and perform Bhastrika to activate Kundalini.
Tadagi (Pond / Tank Seal)	Draw the belly backward so as to make it look like a pond.	Not Mentioned.

Manduki (Frog SEal)	Press the tip of the tongue against the palate and swallow the nectar.	Not Mentioned.
Shambhavi (Shiva's Seal)	Fixing the gaze between the eye-brows, meditate in the Atman.	Not Mentioned as part of 10 Mudra but is later explained in the Samadhi chapter.
Pancha-Dharna (Five Concentration Seal)	Dharna is the process of concentration as mentioned in PYS. Pancha Dharna is concentrating on five different objects. **The details are mentioned below this table.**	Not Mentioned.
Ashwini Mudra (Dawn-Horse Seal)	Contract and relax the anal muscles again and again.	Not Mentioned.
Pashini Mudra (Bird-Catcher SEal)	Throw both legs on the back of the neck and hold them tight as making a noose.	Not Mentioned.

Kaki Mudra (Crow Seal)	One should slowly take in air through the mouth formed like the beak of a crow.	Not Mentioned.
Matangi Mudra (Elephant Seal)	Stand in neck-deep water, draw in water through the two nostrils, and throw it out through the mouth. Then draw in the water through the mouth, and throw it out through the nostrils.	Not Mentioned.
Bhujangini Mudra (Serpent Seal)	Protruding the mouth a little, let one take in air through the throat. (In some books this is shown to be done in Vajrasana or Sukhasana. and in some books, it is shown to be done in Bhujangasana.)	Not Mentioned.

Pancha- Dharna- A collection of 5 mudras referred to as Pancha Dharana.

1. **Parthivi /Adho Dharana-** Element - Earth, Deity- Brahma
   Practice- Think of the earth element in your heart and hold prana along with the Chitta for 2 hours. By Adho-Dharana one can conquer the earth.
2. **Ambhasi Dharana-** Element - Water, Deity- Vishnu
   Practice- Merge Prana and Chitta for 2 hours on the water. This would bring an end to unbearable suffering and sins.
3. **Vaishvnari Dharana-** Element - Fire, Deity- Rudra
   Practice- Merge Prana and Chitta for 2 hours on the fire, which is situated at the navel. This would destroy the terrible dread of death.
4. **Vayavi Dharana-** Element- Air, Deity- Ishwara, Beeja Mantra- Yam
   Practice- Merge Prana and Chitta for 2 hours on the Vayu. This gives the self-restrained aspirants the experience of flying in the air.
5. **Nabho Dharana-** Element- Ether, Deity- Sada-Shiva, Beeja Mantra- Ham
   Practice- Merge Prana and Chitta for 2 hours on the Space / Vyom. This is capable of breaking open the door to liberation.

Chapter 4- Pratyahar

- Pratyahara is the practice of voluntary withdrawal of the sense organs from the sense objects.
- Sage Gherand says that the mind should be withdrawn from what is being seen, heard, felt, tasted, and smelled. Meaning the utmost control of five sense organs or panch-indriyan.

Chapter 5- Pranayama

In this chapter Sage Gherand also talks about how the yogi should live, the best times to practice, the prescribed and prohibited foods for the Yogi, etc.

Prescribed and Prohibited Time

Hemante - Shishire - Greeshme - Varshayam - cha- Ritau - Tatha || Yogarambham - Na - Kurveet - Krate - Yogo - hi - Rogdah || GS 5.8||

Meaning- One should not begin the practice of Yoga in Hemant, Shishir, Grishma, and Varsha Ritu. If practiced yoga causes sickness.

Vasante - Sharadi - Proktam - Yoga - arambham - samacharet ||

Tada - Yogi - Bhavet-Siddho-Roganmukto - Bhavet – Dhruvam || GS 5.9||

Meaning- It is said that one should begin the practice of Yoga in Vasanta and Sharad. Thereby the yogi attains success and verily he becomes free from diseases.

Prescribed Food (Pathya Bhojan)

Shalay - Annam - Yava- Pishtam - Va - Tatha - Godhum - Pishtakam ||

Mudgam-Maschank- Adi - Shubhram - Cha-Tusham-Varjitam || GS 5.17||

Meaning- A yogi should eat food prepared from **rice** (Shalay), **barley flour** (Yava Pishtam), **wheat flour** (Godhuma), **green**

gram (Mudgam), **black gram** etc. which should be cleaned (Shubhram) and free from the husk.

Patolam - Suranam - Manam- kakkolam - cha - Shukshakam ||

dradhikam-karkateem- rambham-dumbarim- kantkantakam ||GS 5.18||

Aamrambham - Balrambham - Rambhadandam - cha - moolkam ||

Vartakeem - Moolkam - Riddhim - Yogi - Bhakshnam – Achret ||GS 5.19||

Meaning- A yogi should eat food **Patolak** (Small Cucumber), **Surana** (Jackfruit), Mana, Kakkola, Sukasaka, Dradhika, Karkati, Rambha, Dumbari, Kantakantake, Amarambha, Balarambha, Rambhandana, Mulaka, Vartak, and Riddhi.

Note: (The meaning of these vegetables are not clear)

Balshakam - Kalshakam - Tatha - Patolakpatram ||

Panchashakam - Prashanseeyat - Vastukam - himlochikam||GS 5.20||

Meaning- Yogi should eat five recommended leafy vegetables- Balsaka, Kalasaka, Patolak-patraka, Vastuka and Himlochika.

Prohibited Food (Apathya Bhojan)

Katu - amlam - lavanam - tiktam - bhrashtam - cha - dadhi - takra-kam ||

Shakotkatam - tatha - madyam-talam-cha-pansam-tatha || GS 5.23||

Kulatham - masuram - pandum - kushmandam - shakdandam ||

Tumbikol - kapittham - cha - kantbilvam - palashkam || GS 5.24||

Kadambam - Jambeeram - Bimbam - Lakucham - Lashunam - Visham|

Kamrangam - Piyalam - Cha - Hingu - Shalmali – Kemukam ||GS 5.25||

Meaning- (In the same order as shloka) Yogis should avoid bitter, sour, salt, pungent, scorched food, curd, buttermilk, too many mixed vegetables, liquor, palm nuts, jackfruits, kulattha, masura, pandu, kusmanda, vegetable-stem, gourds, berries, Kapittha, Kanta-bilva, Palasaka, Kadamba, Jambira, Bimba, Lakuca, Lasuna, Lotus-stalk fibers, Kamaranga, Piyala, Hingu, Salmali, Kemuka.

- Yogi should avoid early morning baths, fasting, etc., or anything that causes fatigue. Similarly, he should **avoid** eating once a day, not eating at all, or eating again within three hours.
- Following these rules, one should practice Pranayama. In the beginning, he should take milk and ghee daily and food twice a day, once at noon and once in the evening.
- He should sit on a thick seat of Kush grass, antelope skin, tiger skin, or a blanket facing the **east or north**. Having purified the Nadis, he should practice Pranayama.

- Then he explains the practice of Nadi-Shodhan Pranayama. (The practice is explained in chapter 1.12)
- He mentions three milestones on the path of pranayama-
  - **The highest type** of pranayama has is Poorak lasting for 20 matras, Kumbhak 80 matras and Rechak for 40 matras.
  - **The moderate** pranayama has Poorak of 16 matra, Kumbhak of 64 matra and Rechak of 32 matra.
  - **The lowest** pranayama has Poorak of 12 matras, Kumbhak of 48 matras, and Rechak of 24 matra
- Based on these 3 stages one goes through different experiences-
  - **The lowest type** of pranayama gives warmth.
  - **The moderate** one gives rise to tremors, particularly in the spinal column.
  - While the **highest type** of pranayama leads to levitation.

After Nadi Shodhan he explains **8 types** of Kumbhakas. These are-

Sahita, Kevali, SuryaBheda- (Same as HYP), **Ujjayi** (Same as HYP), **Sheetali** (Same as HYP), **Bhastrika** (Same as HYP), **Bhramari** (Same as HYP), **Moorchha** (Same as HYP),

Sahita Kumbhaka- Sahita Kumbhaka is said to be of **two kinds-**

Sagarbha and Nigarbha

- **Sagarbha Kumbhaka-**This is performed while **repeating the beej mantra.** It's basically Nadi Shodhan, with chanting OM.
  - Sit in Sukhasana facing east or north, contemplate on Brahma characterized by the letter A and inhale by the left nostril repeating A 16 times.

- Then contemplate on Hari characterized by the letter U perform Kumbhaka repeating U 64 times.
- Then contemplating on Shiva, characterized by the letter M exhale through the right nostril, repeating M 32 times.
- Then again, inhale through the right, retain and exhale through the left in the same way.

- **Nigarbha Kumbhak** - This is performed without mantra repetition.

Kevali Kumbhaka

- Drawing in the air by both nostrils, just stop breathing. On the first day retain breath from 1-64 times.
- One should perform kevali 8 times a day, once every 3 hours or one may do it 5 times a day. First in the early morning, then at noon, then in the evening, then at midnight, and then in the fourth quarter of the night. Or one may do it thrice a day dividing the day into three equal parts, every 8 hours.

Chapter- 6 (Dhyan)

Dhyan is said to be of **three kinds- Sthoola** (Gross), **Jyoti** (Of Light), and **Sookshma** (Subtle).

Sthoola Dhyan- To be done on a concrete image.

Jyoti /Tejo Dhyan- To be done on a mass of light

Sookshma Dhyan- Subtle Dhyan. Yogi performs Shambhavi Mudra to awaken the Kundalini.

Tejodhyan (Jyoti Dhyan) is 100 times superior to Sthoola Dhyana. Sookshma Dhyan, which is the greatest of all is a hundred thousand times superior to Tejodhyan.

Chapter - 7 (Samadhi)

The text explains **6 Types** of samadhi-

Dhyan Samadhi (Meditation samadhi)- This is accomplished by **Shambhavi Mudra.**

Nada Samadhi (Sound samadhi)- This is accomplished by **Bhramari**

Rasanand Samadhi (Bliss in taste)-This is accomplished by Khechari

Laya Samadhi (Absorption)- This is accomplished by Yoni Mudra

Bhakti Yog Samadhi -This is accomplished by devotion and contemplation of one's diety.

Rajyog Samadhi - Also known as Unmani Avastha or Sahajavastha samadhi. This is attained by **Manomoorcha mudra** (Trance).

2.9 Concept Of Nadi

Nadi

Nadi is a subtle mechanism similar to veins and arterial mechanisms. These are the thousands of fine, wire-like structures. which is invisible to the eyes. Through Nadi, prana flows. As mentioned in Varaha Upanishad that the Nadis penetrate the body from the soles of the feet to the crown of the head. In them is Prana, the breath of life.

All the nadis **originate** from one of two centers; Either from the **Kandasthan (a space little below the navel) or from the Heart.**

On the physical level, the nadis correspond to the nervous system but their influence extends beyond this to the astral and spiritual planes of our existence.

Different texts have given different numbers of Nadis. Such as-

- Shiv Samhita says there are 350,000 Nadi.
- Prapanchsar Tantra says there are - 300,000 Nadi.
- Goraksha Satarka - 72,000

Out of these, 3 nadis are of the utmost significance- **Ida, Pingala, and Sushumna.**

Ida- Ida Nadi is connected to the left nostril. It is linked to the right hemisphere of the brain and corresponds to the parasympathetic nervous system. This represents the feminine aspect of a human being and is related to creativity, mental work, coolness, and surrender, and is represented by the moon.

Pingala- Pingala Nadi is connected to the right nostril. It is linked to the left hemisphere of the brain and corresponds to the sympathetic nervous system. This represents the masculine aspect of a human being and is related to execution, physical work, and heat, and is represented by the sun.

Sushumna- Through Hatha, a balance between these two (Ida and Pingala) can be achieved which then activates a very significant Nadi called Sushumna. Sushumna is found in the spinal cord and has 3 more layers within it. The outer surface of the middle Nadi is Sushumna, inside that is Vajra Nadi, within that Chitrani, and in the very center there is Brahma Nadi

- Sushumna nadi is associated with Tamo Guna
- Vajra Nadi is associated with Rajo Guna; Dynamism.
- Chitrani is associated with Satva Guna
- Brahma Nadi is associated with the unconditioned state of consciousness.

Pingala is referred as Ganga, Ida as Yamuna, and Sushumna as Saraswati.

Impurities of Nadis

Gherand Samhita says that when Nadi is full of impurities, Vayu does not enter them. These impurities are waste and residue of sensuous living and desires. Just as excess fat accumulates around blood vessels and can eventually obstruct the blood flow, similarly on a pranic level there is an accumulation of waste. With the build-up of this waste body's capacity to circulate energy lessens. The body becomes lethargic, the energy level decreases, and activation of the chakras and higher brain function is prevented.

If Kundalini is released when the Nadis are blocked and weak, sadhak will not be able to handle the experience. For the ultimate experience, the whole body, the network of Nadi along with the energy channels have to be made strong.

The Pranic body (Pranayama Kosha) is the intermediate link between the Physical sheath (Annamaya Kosha) and the Mind sheath (Manomaya Kosha). Hence it can be approached from either side. It can be easier to control and purify the Pranayama Kosha through the Annamaya Kosha.

By strengthening the sympathetic and parasympathetic nervous system (through asana, pranayama, and Shatkriyas) Ida and Pingala Nadi are affected, and through CNS, Sushumna can be activated.

Concept of Alternate Rhinitis (Swara)

We do not always breathe through both nostrils. The breath alternates from Ida to Pingala every 60 to 90 minutes. In Yoga, this is called Swara.

Modern science affirms this phenomenon and calls it **Alternate Rhinitis**. The Cerberus alternates its activities every 60-90 minutes as indicated by the nostril functions. When the breath is flowing through the left nostril it indicates that Ida and the right brain hemisphere are active and when it flows through the right nostril it means Pingala and the left-brain hemisphere are active.

According to Swara Yog during the flow of Ida, one should do the quiet tasks and those requiring mental creativity, and during the flow of Pingala physical work should be done. The flow of Sushumna (Both the nadis together) is the most suitable time for productive activity and for Yoga Abhyasa and Dhyana.

Nadi Shodhan Pranayama brings the balance between Ida and Pingala Nadi.

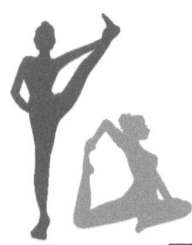

UNIT 3

INTRODUCTION TO YOGA TEXT

3.1 General introduction to the human body and nine major systems of the human body-

The human body shows a unique organizational unity that aids in carrying out activities in a synchronized and integrated manner. Let's understand the structure of the human body.

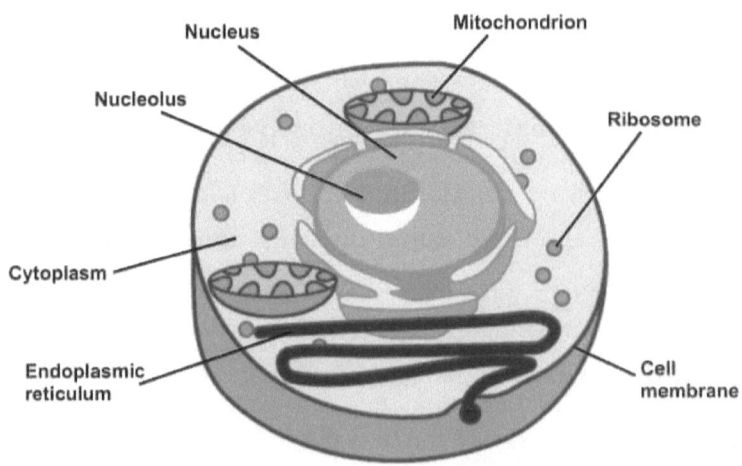

Cell- This is the smallest independently functioning unit of all organisms. A cell contains Mitochondrion, Cytoplasm, Ribosomes, Cell membrane, Nucleus etc. Mitochondria is **the powerhouse of energy.**

Tissue- The cells that form a separate specialized group are coined as tissue.

Organ- Various kinds of tissues come together to create various organs. Such as abdomen, heart, lungs etc.

Organ system- A group of organs that work together to carry out a particular function. Such as Digestive system, Cardiovascular system, Respiratory system etc.

Organism- A living being that has a cellular structure and that can independently perform all physiological functions necessary for life.

It is important to understand that the body function is a collective working of all the cells which make the body. The proper working of every single cell is the most essential factor for the body's survival.

There are 9 major body systems / organ system

Skeletal System, Muscular System, Nervous System, Endocrine System, Respiratory System, Cardiac System, Digestive System, Excretory System, Reproductive System

Musculoskeletal System

The musculoskeletal system refers to skeletal and muscular system in the body. It provides support, stability, shape, and movement to the body. It consists of bones, muscles, joints, cartilage, and connective tissues such as Tendons and Ligaments.

Skeletal System

Bones- There are 206 bones in the human body. These are the main mineral reservoirs. They store calcium and phosphate and release them according to the body's needs.

- Red bone marrow is the body's production center of red blood cells such as vertebrae, ribs, breastbone, and pelvis.
- Muscles are connected to bones by tendons.
- Bones are held together by Ligaments.

Classification of Bones

Long Bones- Responsible for most body movements such as **Femur** (Thigh Bones; largest bone,) **Tibia, Fibula** (Calf bone), etc.

Short Bones- Provide limited motion such as - **Stapes** (Middle ear; smallest bone), **Patella** (Knee cap), **Tarsals** (foot bone), and **Carpal** (hand bone).

Flat Bones- These protect internal organs. such as - **Skull, Thoracic cage**, etc.

Irregular Bones- These have complex shapes and help protect internal organs. Irregular bones of the vertebral column, protect the spinal cord. The irregular bones of the **pelvis (Pubis, ilium, and ischium)** protect organs in the pelvic cavity.

The human skeleton is divided into 2 parts- **Axial Skeleton and Appendicular Skeleton**

Axial Skeleton- This comprises skull bones, vertebral column, and thoracic cage.

- **Skull Bones- (22 Flat Bones)** - There are 2 major parts of the skull
  - **Cranial Bones- (8)** These protect the brain. These bones are connected by Sutures.
  - **Facial Bones- (14)** These give structure to the face

- **Vertebral Columns- (26 irregular bones)-** The Spine can be divided into 5 sections.
  - **Cervical Vertebrae-** C1-C7
  - **Thoracic Vertebrae-** T1-T12
  - **Lumbar Vertebrae-** L1-L5
  - **Sacrum-** 5 vertebrae fused together.
  - **Coccyx** (Tailbone)- 4 bones fused together

- **Thoracic Cage-** This consists of the **sternum, ribs, and a lot of costal cartilage.**
  - **Sternum-** (3 small bones fused together)-This is a flat bone in the middle of the thoracic and it is made of 3 smaller bones that are fused together.
  - **Ribs-** There are 12 pairs of ribs that project from the vertebrae. These can be categorized into 3 categories-
  - **True Ribs (1-7)-** These are called true ribs as they are directly attached to the sternum via costal cartilages.
  - **False Ribs (8-10)-** These are attached indirectly to the sternum via costal cartilages from the ribs above.
  - **Floating Ribs (11-12)** These are called floating ribs as they don't attach to the sternum at all.

Appendicular Skeleton- This consists of **Pectoral Girdle, The Upper Limbs, The Lower Limbs, and The Pelvic Girdle.**

- **Pectoral Girdle-** This consists of the **clavicle** (collar bone) and **scapula** (shoulder bone) which together give structure to the shoulder.
- **The upper limbs-** The upper limbs are **arms, forearms, and hands.**
    - **Arm-** In the arm, there is a "**Humor**" bone.
    - **Forearm-** In the forearm, there is **Ulna and Radius** bone
    - **Hand- (8+5+14 = 27)-** The wrist is made up of 8 short bones called **Carpals**. The palms are made of 5 bones called **Metacarpals**. The finger bones are called **Phalanges** and are 14 in number.
- **The lower limbs-** This consists of the **thigh, calf, and foot**.
    - **Thigh-** The thigh has the largest bone in the body called **Femur.**
    - **Calf-** The calf contains 2 bones **Tibia and Fibula**.
    - **Foot (7+5+14)-** 7 **Tarsals**, 5 **Metatarsals**, and 14 **Phalanges**.
- **Pelvic Girdle-** Pelvic girdle starts at the sacrum and continues with 2 hip bones. These 2 hip bones are actually made of 3 separate bones- **Ilium, Ischium, and Pubis.**

Connective Tissues- These are the tissues that help to connect all the organs and parts of the body.

- Tissues that connect **2 bones** are called **Ligaments.**
- Tissues that connect **muscle to the bone** are called **Tendon**
- Tissues that connect **2 muscles** are called **Fascia.**

Joint- This is a connection b/w **2 bones** in a human skeleton. Joints can be classified by - **Structure, Mobility, and Range of Motion.**

Classification of joint as per structure- There are 3 types of joints-

1. **Synovial Joint-** These are called Synovial joints as there is Synovial fluid in these joints. There are **6 synovial joints** in the body.

- **Ball and Socket Joints-** It is a polyaxial joint that gives the most range of motion and movements. The movements of these joints are Flexion, Extension, Adduction, Abduction, Internal rotation, and External Rotation. Such as - Hip joint, Shoulder joint.
- **Hinge Joints-** It is a uniaxial joint with only flexion and extension movements. Such as - Knee joint, Elbow Joint.
- **Pivot Joint-** It is a uniaxial joint that allows movements on a single axis. The movement of this joint is Rotation. Such as 1. The joint of the first and the second cervical vertebrae (Atlas and Axis), allows for the turning of the head from side to side. 2. The joint of the wrist that allows the palm of the hand to be turned up and down.
- **Condyloid Joint-** This is a biaxial joint, which means it allows movement into 2 axes. The movements are Radial Deviation and Ulnar Deviation, Flexion, and Extension. Such as Wrist Joints.
- **Saddle Joint-** The movements of this joint are Abduction, Adduction, Flexion, Extension, and Circumduction. Such as- Thumb

- **Plane / Gliding Joint**- Example- Shoulder and Hip Joint.

2. **Fibrous Joint**- These are bound by tough fibrous connective tissue. These joints exhibit little to no mobility. These can be divided into 3 types-

- **Suture**- This joint is found exclusively b/w the bones of the skull.
- **Gomphosis**- This is found in teeth.
- **Syndesmosis**- This is bound by ligaments. such as- Forearm

3. **Cartilaginous Joint**- In this type of joint bones are joined by Hyaline Cartilage. These are of 2 types-

- **Synchondroses**- These are also known as Primary cartilaginous joint
- **Symphyses**- This is a secondary cartilaginous joint. This is found along the midline of the body.

Muscular System

This is made up of over 600 muscles. These can be divided into 3 categories-

Cardiac Muscle- This is an **involuntary** muscle. These muscles form the walls of the heart and contract to circulate the blood. These have a striped appearance and are also categorized as **Striated** Muscles.

Visceral / Smooth Muscle- These are **involuntary** muscles. These are found in organs or organ systems such as the digestive system, respiratory system, etc. These are **non-striated** muscles.

Skeletal Muscles- These are **voluntary** muscles. These are attached to the skeleton and provide the skeleton with the ability to move. These are also of **Striated** Type.

There are 5 types of basic muscle movements- **Adduction, Abduction, Flexion, Extension, and Rotation**

Respiratory System-

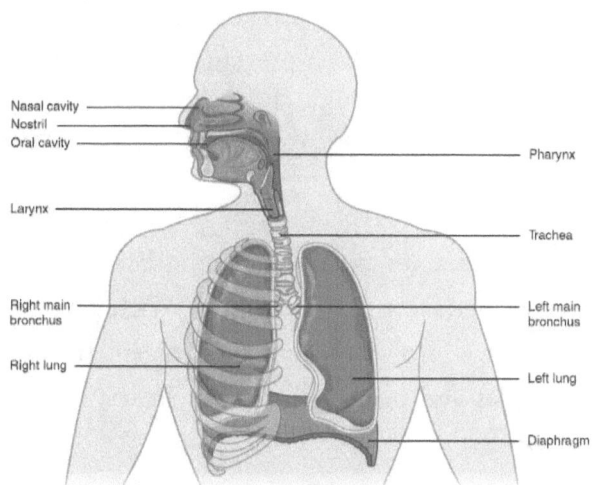

The human respiratory system has 2 parts.

Upper Respiratory System- This consists of the Nasal cavity, Pharynx, Larynx (Voice Box)

Lower Respiratory System- This consists of Trachea, Brachia, Bronchioles, and lungs.

In humans, the main organs responsible for breathing are present in the thoracic cavity. These are dome-shaped fibrous tissue known as Diaphragm and lungs.

Right Lung- This is divided into 3 lubes; **Right Superior, Right Middle, and Right Inferior Lube.**

Left Lung- This is smaller and has only 2 lubes. **Left Superior and Left Inferior.**

Bronchi- Both the lungs are associated externally with small tubular Bronchi which unite and extend into the Trachea.

Trachea- The Trachea is a tube-like structure that connects the larynx to the bronchi of the lungs. The trachea has incomplete 'C' shaped rings of cartilage which prevents the Tracheal wall from collapsing. Trachea leads to the pharynx, which is connected to the nostrils.

As we breathe in the oxygen moves downwards through the pharynx and trachea, to finally reach the Bronchi. From each Bronchus oxygen travels into the lungs. Within the lungs, the Bronchus divides into Bronchioles. Oxygen travels through these Bronchioles and reaches to alveoli. **In the Alveoli** the gas exchange happens.

VC- The maximal volume of air that can be exhaled after maximum inhalation is referred to as Vital Capacity.

LV- Lung volumes are also known as respiratory volumes. It refers to the volume of gas in the lungs at a given time during the respiratory cycle. The average total lung volume/ capacity of an adult human male is about 6 liters of air.

MVV- The largest amount of air that a person can inhale and then exhale during a 12- to 15-s interval with maximal voluntary effort is referred to as Maximum Voluntary Ventilation Capacity.

FVC- Forced vital capacity is the amount of air that can be forcibly exhaled from your lungs after taking the deepest breath possible.

Cardiovascular System

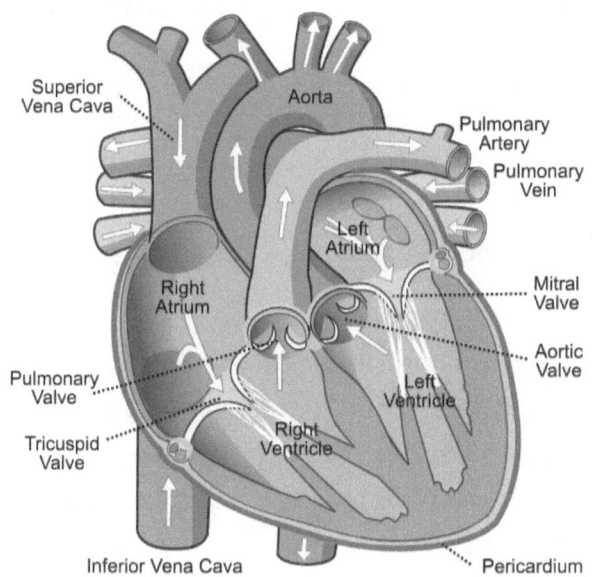

The cardiovascular system is part of the **circulatory system** which circulates blood. The circulatory system also includes the Lymphatic system which circulates Lymph.

Cardiovascular System + Lymphatic System Circulatory System.

Cardiovascular systems consist of the Heart, Blood, and Blood vessels.

Heart- This essentially is a pump that moves blood through the vessels. It has 2 sides, each of which has 2 chambers. The upper part has the **Right Atrium and Left Atrium**, and the lower part has the **Right Ventricle and Left Ventricle**.

The beating heart contracts and relaxes. Contraction is called **Systole** and relaxation is called **Diastole**. The best-known function of the circulatory system is the transport of inhaled oxygen from the lungs to the body's tissues and the removal of CO_2 in the opposite direction.

Through the **Vena Cova veins (Largest Veins)**, oxygen-poor blood returns to the **RA** (Right Atrium) and then to **RV** (Right Ventricle), and from there, it is pumped to the lungs through the **Pulmonary Artery**. In the lungs, the blood picks up **O_2 and releases CO_2**.

The **oxygen-rich blood** returns to the **LA** (Left Atrium) and then to the **LV** (Left Ventricle). From here it gets pumped into the body's tissue through the Aorta **(Largest Artery)** Where it unlocks oxygen and picks up CO_2. The resulting de-oxygenated blood returns to the RA to complete the circuit.

Arteries that feed the oxygen-rich blood to the heart are called **coronary arteries.**

Blood Vessels- Blood vessels are meant to carry blood throughout the body. These are of two types- Arteries and Veins.

- **Oxygenated blood** flows to the body from the heart through the **Arteries. Pulmonary arteries** are the only arteries that carry deoxygenated blood
- The **Deoxygenated blood** flows back from the body to the heart through **the Veins.**
- Capillaries are the smallest blood vessels.

Blood- Blood is a fluid made of plasma. Plasma is **90% water**. Its pH level is usually close to 7.40. There are 3 types of blood cells - **Erythrocytes** / Red Blood Cells, **Leukocytes** / White Blood Cells, and **Thrombocytes** / Platelets.

Blood Pressure is the force that the heart uses to pump blood in the body. It is measured in the unit of millimeters of mercury (mmHg). The instrument is called **Sphygmomanometer**

Systolic Pressure is the pressure the heart uses to push the blood out. **Diastolic Pressure** is the pressure when the heart rest between beats, hence a BP reading of 140/90 mmHg means, Systolic pressure of 140 mmHg and Diastolic pressure of 90 mmHg. **The ideal BP reading** is considered between 90/60 mmHg - 120/80 mmHg.

Anemia is a condition of not having enough healthy red blood cells in the body. This condition is usually caused by a lack of Iron, Vitamin B12 (Cobalamin), and Folate deficiency.

Imp- The pH level of drinking water lies b/w 6.5-8.5.

Nervous System

The basic purpose of the nervous system is to

Coordinate all activities of the body along with enabling the body to respond and adapt to changes both inside and out.

The **basic unit** of communication in the nervous system is called **neurons.**

The nervous system is split into 2 parts- the **Central Nervous System**, and the **Peripheral Nervous System**

Central Nervous System (CNS)-This is made up of the **brain and Spinal Cord.**

Brain- The brain is found within the cranium and has 6 major sections.

- **Cerebrum-** This is the largest section of the brain which is divided into the right and left brain hemispheres. This is further divided into 4 lobes.
    o **Frontal** - Responsible for reasoning and thoughts.
    o **Parietal-** Integrates sensory information.
    o **Temporal-** Processes auditory information from the ears.
    o **Occipital-** Processing visual information from the eyes.
- **Cerebellum-** Located at the back of the head, This is responsible for muscle coordination, maintaining balance and posture, and coordinating eye movements
- **Diencephalon-** This section is found b/w the cerebrum and the midbrain, It contains 2 structures.
    o **Thalamus-** It behaves like a relay station and directs sensory impulses to the cerebrum.
    o **Hypothalamus-** This structure controls and regulates temperature, appetite, water balance, sleep, and blood vessel constriction and dilation. Hypothalamus also plays a role in emotions such as Anger, Fear. Pleasure, Pain, and Affection.
- **Midbrain-** This is located below the cerebrum at the top of the brain stem. It is responsible for eyes and auditory reflexes.
- **Pons-** This is located below the midbrain into the brainstem. It is responsible for certain reflex actions such as chewing, tasting, and salivary production.

- **Medulla Oblongata-** This is located at the bottom of the brainstem and connects to the spinal cord. This is responsible for heart and blood vessel function, Swallowing, Coughing, Sneezing, Blood-Pressure, Digestion, and Respiration; This is also known as the **center of respiration,**

Spinal Cord- The spinal cord is the link b/w the brain and the nerves in the rest of the body. The spinal cord has different sections. These are- Cervical (C1-C7), Thoracic (T1-T12), Lumbar (L1-L5), Sacrum, and Coccyx. The Spinal cord is connected to the body through 2 types of Spinal Nerves- Afferent and Efferent

- **Afferent nerves** carry information from the body to the brain
- **Efferent nerves** carry information from the brain to the body.

Peripheral Nervous System (PNS)- This is the nervous system outside the brain and spinal cord. This is further divided into 2 types.

1. **Somatic Nervous System-** The somatic nervous system is responsible for carrying motor and sensory information.. This system is responsible for nearly all voluntary muscle movements as well as processes sensory information from external stimulation such as hearing, touch, and sight.

The **Afferent neurons** take information **from the nerves** to the CNS and the **Efferent neurons** take information **from the CNS** to the muscle fibers throughout the body.

2. **The Autonomic Nervous System** (ANS)- This is further divided into the Sympathetic and Parasympathetic Nervous Systems.

- **The Sympathetic Nervous System** - This is essential for our survival. This nervous system revs up the body to either defend yourself or escape the threat; called **Fight or Flight Response**. This is located near the Thoracic and Lumbar regions in the Spinal cord
- **The Parasympathetic Nervous System**- This system brings all systems of the body back to normal once the threat is gone. This is known as the **"Rest and Digest"** or **"Feed and Breed"** response. This system is located between the spinal cord and the medulla.

Digestive System

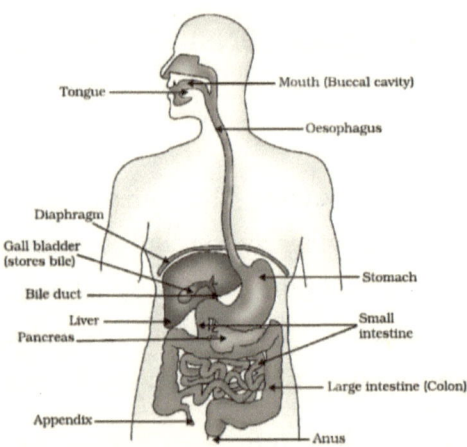

The digestive system includes organs that break food down into the protein, vitamins, minerals, fats, and carbs which are required by the body for energy, growth, and repair. The digestive system is divided into 2 parts. -

1. **Alimentary canal / Gastrointestinal Tract-** This is **one long tube** that extends from the **mouth to Anus**. This tract consists of the mouth, esophagus, stomach, small intestine, large intestine, and anus. Hence it is a series of hollow organs joined in a long, twisting tube from the mouth to the anus.
2. **Accessory Digestive System-** These are the organs that help in digestion but are not part of the digestive tract. The 5 accessory digestive organs are the **Tongue, Salivary Glands, Pancreas, Liver, and Gallbladder.**

The main actions which take place in this system are-

Ingestion- Chewing, **Propulsion-** Swallowing, food movement through peristalsis, **Mechanical Breakdown-** Churning in the stomach, **Segmentation, Digestion, Absorption, Defecation.**

> **Peristalsis** is a function of ANS (Parasympathetic Nervous System). Peristalsis movements predominate in the esophagus, whereas the **Segmentation** contraction occurs in the large and small intestines.

Organs of Digestive System

Mouth-

- The process of digestion begins from the mouth.
- The organs which help in chewing the food are - **Tongue, Teeth, and Palate.**

Salivary Gland- The mouth receives the secretion from the salivary glands- **The parotid gland, submandibular gland, and sublingual gland.** Saliva contains 2 important enzymes

- **Amylase**- breaks starch into simple sugar, and **Lipase**- breaks fats into simple lipids.
- Once the food is chewed it makes its way through the pharynx into the esophagus.
- **The epiglottis** is a piece of cartilage that covers the opening of the "Larynx".
- When we breathe, the epiglottis is open and the air is passed down the "trachea" while eating, the epiglottis is closed. so, the larynx opening gets closed and food enters the esophagus.

Esophagus- This is a **25 cm long** muscular tube of smooth muscles through which food passes into the stomach due to **peristalsis.**

At the lower end of the esophagus (where it connects with the stomach) there is a **"cardiac sphincter"**. These are very strong muscles and remain constricted at all times to prevent the acid from the stomach from moving upwards in the esophagus. Only when we eat, do these muscles relax to give one-way movement to the food i.e. into the stomach.

Stomach- This is a "J" shaped organ that is connected to the "esophagus" at the upper end and the "Duodenum" at the lower end.

The stomach has smooth muscles in arrangements of layers that turn the stomach into a churner. These are - **Mucosa, Sub-mucosa, Muscle Layer, and Serosa.** Out of these, Mucosa is the innermost layer, and Serosa is the outermost layer.

Muscle layers cause the waves of powerful contraction (Peristalsis) which cause the mechanical churning of food.

The stomach releases strong chemicals like **HCL, NACL, and Pepsinogen** (This enzyme digests protein). Since these chemicals can harm the stomach wall, a "mucus" which is secreted by gastric glands protects the stomach wall.

The lower part of the stomach is called the **"PYLORUS"**. This also has a strong smooth muscle sphincter which is called the **"Pyloric Sphincter"**. The Pyloric sphincter opens one hour after taking the meal. By this time the meal gets converted into a semi-liquid called **"Chyme"**

Small Intestine- This is a **5 M long tube** that is divided into 3 parts- **Duodenum (25 cm long), Jejunum (The curled part), and ileum (The lower part)**. The small intestine has the main function of digestion and absorption of the food. The enzymes from the liver, pancreas, gallbladder, and intestinal wall itself, together do the task.

Most of the digestion happens in the small intestine. Through Segmental contraction, food moves forward slowly. The main enzymes which react to proteins (amino acids) are Pancreatic enzymes Chymotrypsinogen and Trypsin.

The intestinal wall has a small hair-like structure called **'Villi'**. These villi even have microstructures on them called microvilli. This mechanism increases the surface area of the small intestine.

Liver- The liver is a vital organ of the digestive system which releases **"Bile"** which helps in fat digestion. Bile contains **97% water**, Bile salt, Bile pigments, and mucus. These secretions are received in the Duodenum, through the "Bile Duct". Gall

Bladder stores "Bile" and concentrates it. It is the largest gland in the body

Pancreas- The pancreas has both **endocrines as well as exocrine Glands**. The endocrine part primarily releases **Insulin and Glucagon**, and the Exocrine part primarily produces digestive juices.

Large Intestine- This is a **1.5 M long tube** that is divided into **Ascending, Transverse, and Descending colons.** The food which is not digested passes through the large intestine. This begins with **"Ceacum"** which marks the distinction b/w small and large colons.

The descending colon leads to the **"Sigmoid Colon"** which then leads to the rectum which leads to the anal canal. The large intestine contains almost 700 types of bacteria.

Gland System

Glands are organs that secrete substances into the body for use or discharge. There are two types of glands - **Endocrine and Exocrine.**

Endocrine- The endocrine glands are **ductless glands**. Their secretion is directly absorbed into the blood. This system makes Hormones. such as - **Pituitary, Thyroid, Adrenal, etc.**

Exocrine- These are **duct glands**. Their secretion is first stored in these ducts and then gets released upon specific stimulation. These are non- hormonal glands, and usually secret fluids like tears, sweat, etc. Such As- **Mammary Gland, Salivary Gland,**

Sudoriferous (sweat gland), Sebaceous (oil gland), and Lacrimal gland (Tear gland).

Endocrine System- Modern endocrinology originated in the 20th century from the work of a French physiologist **"Claude Bernard"**.

Claude Bernard made a key observation that the human body maintains a constant internal environment which he termed a **"Milieu Interior"**. He observed that this Milieu Interior is preserved by various systems of the body such as the nervous system, and immune system along with a set of glands that secrete "Hormones", i.e., Chemical messengers.

The human body needs control over its cells, tissue, and various processes in the body so that it can function in an orderly and stable way which makes vital functions like growth, development, and reproduction possible.

This control is provided by 3 functions in the body - **Nervous System, Immune System, and Endocrine System.**

The nervous system is in charge of various body processes which happen rather fast such as movements, breathing, etc. **The immune system** is responsible for actions against damage, illness, etc. **The endocrine system**, in general, is in charge of the body's processes which happen rather slowly. Such as The rate of height increase, maintenance of electrolytes and ions in the blood, the Body's metabolic rate, etc

How does the endocrine system work?

Various endocrine glands sense the various processes in the body and receive the necessary stimuli as a reaction. Upon receiving that, these glands secrete hormones that act as chemical messengers which then get distributed to the whole of the body to initiate a special effect.

Such as- Pancreas secretes "Insulin" which is a hormone that regulates blood sugar levels. Let's see how this really happens-

The pancreas has a rich blood supply through which it senses the blood glucose concentration. Whenever we eat, the glucose level in the blood rises which is detected by the pancreas. Upon this detection, the pancreas releases "insulin". This Hormone activates most of the cells in the body to take up the extra sugar. This activity is important to normalize the blood sugar concentration level.

Imp:

- The smallest gland as well as organ in the body is Pineal Gland.
- The largest gland in the body is Liver.
- The largest organ in the body is Skin.

Hormones can usually be divided into 3 categories-

1. **Steroid Hormones-** These are lipophilic (fat loving) meaning they can freely diffuse across the plasma membrane of a cell. Such as Estrogen, Progesterone, Testosterone, TH, FSH, etc.
2. **Peptide Hormones-** These are hydrophilic and lipophobic (fat-hating), meaning they cannot freely cross the plasma

membrane. These bind to the receptors on the surface of the cells. Such as Insulin, Glucagon, Leptin, ADH, and Oxytocin.

3. **Amine Hormone-** These are derived from the amino acid "Tyrosine". Such as Adrenaline, Thyroxine, and Tri-Modo-thyroxine.

Thyroid Gland- (Protein / Amine Hormone)-

This is located immediately below the larynx and is the largest endocrine gland. This weighs 15-20 grams. This secret- **Triiodothyronine (T3)- 7%, and Thyroxine (T4)- 93%.** Thyroid glands require iodine for this synthesis in a dose of 1 mg/week.

Functions- Regulating cell metabolism, and heart rate. It also regulates how fast the intestines process food.

Parathyroid Gland

Parathyroid glands are 4 small glands that are located behind the thyroid. These are responsible for continuously monitoring and regulating blood calcium levels. Calcium is the only element with its own regulatory system- "The Parathyroid Glands".

The Role of Calcium in the Human Body

The **prime role** of Calcium is to provide **electrical energy** for the nervous system, muscular system, and skeletal system. Bones are the main reservoir of calcium.

Adrenal Glands / Suprarenal glands

These are called **adrenal** as they are present just **adjacent to the kidneys**. They are also known as supra-renal as they are located above the kidneys. Adrenal glands are triangular-shaped and made up of Cortex and Medulla. The cortex primarily releases hormones such as **Aldosterone, Cortisol, and Androgens.**

The medulla primarily releases hormones such as **Epinephrine (Adrenaline) and Non-Epinephrine (nor-adrenaline).** These hormones are often activated in physically and emotionally stressful situations **(Fight or Flight Response).**

Functions- Increasing the heart rate, Increasing blood flow to the muscle and brain, Assisting in Glucose (Sugar) Metabolism, etc.

Pancreas

This organ consists of both endocrine and exocrine parts.

Exocrine Function- These glands produce enzymes important for digestion. These are -**Trypsin** - To digest protein, **Amylase**- To digest carbs, and **Lipase-** To break down fats.

Endocrine Function- The Endocrine part of the Pancreas contains around 1 million islets which are called **Islets of Langerhans**. This part produces hormones that are necessary for blood sugar control- **Insulin and Glucagon**

Insulin

- Whenever we eat, there is **a rise in blood sugar** concentration which is detected by the pancreas, and Pancreas releases insulin.
- Insulin acts as a **Key** to open up the cells in the body and allows glucose to be used as an energy source.
- Additionally, when there is excess glucose in the bloodstream known as, Insulin encourages the storage of Glucose as **Glycogen in the liver**, muscle, and fat cells.

- These stores can then be used at a later time when energy requirements are higher.
- As a result of this, there is less insulin in the bloodstream, and normal blood glucose levels are restored.
- When the **liver is saturated with glycogen**, an alternative pathway takes over. This involves the uptake of additional glucose into **adipose tissues**. Leading to the synthesis of lipoproteins.
- The liver can store up to **5%** of its mass as glycogen.
- Insulin is an **Anabolic Hormone** as it encourages the formation of glycogen (complex molecule) from glucose (simple molecule). It also prevents the breakdown of fats and proteins.

Absence of Insulin- In the absence of Insulin, the body is not able to utilize glucose as energy in the cells. As a result, the glucose remains in the bloodstream and leads to high blood sugar, known as **Hyperglycaemia and may lead to Type 2 diabetes.**

In severe cases, lack of insulin and reduced ability to use glucose as a source of energy can lead to a reliance on fat stores as the sole source of energy. The breakdown of these fats can release Ketones into the bloodstream, which can lead to a condition called Ketoacidosis. Ketoacidosis is a severe condition that involves symptoms like- Vomiting, Dehydration, An unusual smell on the breath, Deep labored breathing or hyperventilation, Rapid Heartbeat, Confusion and disorientation, etc.

Glucagon- The role of Glucagon is **to prevent** blood glucose levels from dropping too low. This is a **catabolic Hormone** as it stimulates the conversion of stored Glycogen (stored in the liver) to glucose.

Excretory System

The excretory system consists of organs that remove metabolic wastes and toxins from the body such as the **Urinary system, skin, nails, etc.** The primary excretory organs in the human body are the **kidneys, ureters, urethra, and urinary bladder.**

Kidney- The basic functional unit of the Kidney is called **Nephron**. These nephrons perform the primary task of filtering blood and removing waste products.

Ureters- These are pairs of thin muscular tubes that come out of each kidney and carry urine from the kidney to the urinary bladder.

The Urinary Bladder- This is a muscular sac-like structure, which stores urine.

The Urethra- This is a tube that arises from the urinary bladder and helps to expel urine from the body. In males, it also acts as the common route for sperm as well as urine.

Reproductive System

Male Gonads- The testicles (Gonads) are a pair of sperm-producing organs that maintain the health of the male reproductive system. Their female counterparts are Ovaries.

The primary secretion of gonads is **Testosterone** which is vital to the normal development of male physical characteristics. Such as The healthy development of male sex organs, Growth of facial and body hair, Lowering the voice, Increase in height, Increase in muscle mass, Growth of Adam's apple, Maintaining libido, Sperm production, Promoting healthy bone density etc.

Female Gonads

Ovaries- Ovaries secret 2 very important hormones- **Estrogen and Progesterone.**

Estrogen- There are three major estrogens- **Estradiol, Estrone, and Estriol**

Estradiol is instrumental in breast and reproductive organs development, fat distribution in the hips, legs, and breasts etc.

Progesterone- This hormone mainly acts on the uterus cervix and vagina and prepares these organs for **conception.**

3.2 Introduction to sensory organs

(Eyes, Nose, Ears, Tongue, and Skin)

Eyes-

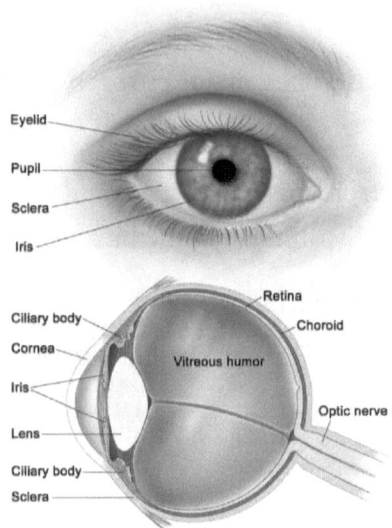

Sight is arguably our most important sense. More of the brain is dedicated to vision than to hearing, taste, touch, and smell combined. Vision is an incredibly complex process that works so well, we never need to give it much thought.

In simple words- Light enters our pupil and is focused onto the retina at the back of the eye. The retina converts the light signal into electrical impulses. The optic nerve then carries the impulses to the brain where the signals are processed.

Anatomy of the eye

The tissues of the eyes can be split into three types- **Refracting tissues**- these focus light, **Light-sensitive tissues**, and **support tissues.**

Refracting Tissues- Refracting tissues focus incoming light onto the light-sensitive tissues, to give us a clear, sharp image. If these are wrongly shaped, misaligned, or damaged, vision can be blurry. The refracting tissues include-

The Pupil- This is the dark spot in the center of the colored part of the eye. The pupil expands and shrinks in response to the light.

Iris- This is the colored portion of the eye. Iris is a muscle that controls the size of the pupil and therefore, the amount of light reaching the retina.

Lens- Once the light has travelled through the pupil, it reaches the lens which is a transparent convex structure. The lens can change shape, helping the eye to focus light accurately onto the retina. With age, the lens becomes stiffer and less flexible, making focusing more difficult.

Ciliary Muscles- This muscular ring is attached to the lens and changes its shape as it contracts or relaxes. This process is called accommodation.

Cornea- This is a transparent dome-like layer that covers the pupil, iris, and anterior chamber or fluid-filled area between the cornea and the iris. It is responsible for the majority of the eye's focusing power. However, it has a fixed focus so cannot adjust to different distances. It is the eye's first defence against foreign objects and injury.

Because the cornea must remain clear to refract light, it has no blood vessels. Two fluids circulate throughout the eyes to provide structure and nutrients, these fluids are- **Vitreous Fluid-** This is found in the back section of the eye. Vitreous Fluid is thick and gel-like. It makes up the majority of the eye's mass.

Aqueous Fluid- This is more watery than vitreous fluid and circulates through the front of the eye.

Light Sensitive Tissues- These include-

Retina- This is the innermost layer of the eye. It houses more than 120 million light-sensitive, photoreceptors cells that detect light and convert it into electrical signals. These signals are sent to the brain for processing. **Photoreceptors cells** in the retina contain protein molecules called **Opsins** that are sensitive to light.

The two primary photoreceptors cells are **rods and cones.**

Cones- These are found in the central region of the retina called the macula. Cones are essential for detailed, color vision.

Rods- These are mostly found around the edges of the retina and are used for seeing in low light levels. Although they cannot distinguish colors, they are extremely sensitive and can detect the lowest amount of light.

Optic Nerve- This is a thick bundle of nerve fibers that transmits signals from the retina to the brain. There are around 1 million thin, retinal fibers called ganglion cells that carry light information from the retina to the brain for processing visual information.

Support Tissues- These include-

Sclera- This is commonly referred to as the white of the eye. It is fibrous and provides support for the eyeball, helping it keep its shape.

Conjunctiva- A thin, transparent membrane that covers most of the white of the eye and the inside of the eyelids. It helps lubricate the eye and protect it from microbes.

Choroid- This is a layer of connective tissue between the retina and sclera. It is just 0.5 mm thick and contains light-absorbing pigment cells that help reduce reflection in the retina.

Nose-

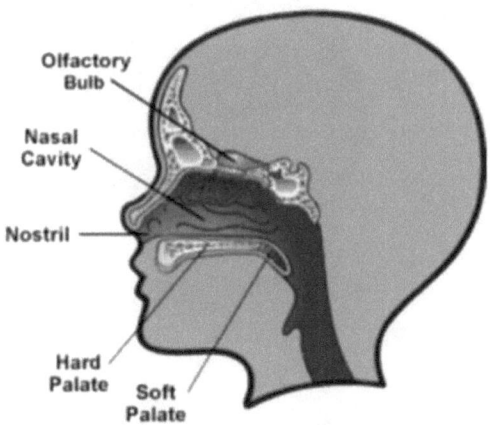

The nose helps in breathing and smelling. It is a hollow air passage that consists of two nasal chambers called nostrils.

The roof of the nose is lined with nerve cells which are responsible for detecting different smells. These cells are connected to the Olfactory bulb which is connected to the Olfactory cortex in the brain. The nose is made up of –

- **External Meatus-** Triangular-shaped projection in the center of the face.
- **External Nostrils-** Two chambers divided by septum.
- **Septum-** Made up mainly of cartilage and bone and covered by mucous membrane.
- **Nasal Passage-** Passages that are lined with mucous membranes and tiny hairs (cilia) that help to filter the air.
- **Sinuses-** Four pairs of air-filled cavities, also lined with mucous membranes.

Tongue-

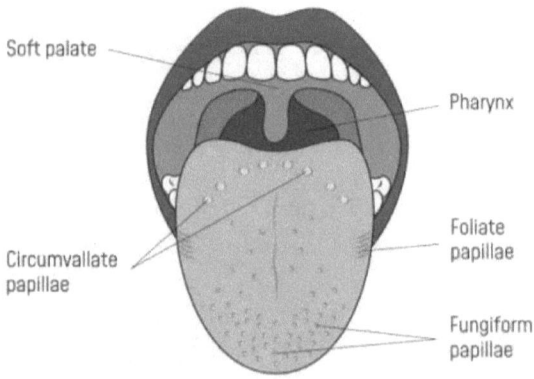

The tongue is a muscular organ in the mouth covered with a moist, pink tissue called the mucosa. It is involved in licking, tasting, breathing, swallowing, and speaking.

The papillae present on the tongue give it a rough texture. It is covered by a number of taste buds. There are several nerves in the tongue that help in transmitting taste signals to the brain and thus helps in taste sensation.

The tongue is divided into the anterior and posterior parts.

The Anterior Part- This is the oral part that includes the root attached to the floor of the oral cavity.

The Posterior Part- This is known as the Pharyngeal or Post Sulcus Part which includes the base forming the ventral wall of the oropharynx.

The tongue is made up of three elements- **Epithelium** (comprised of papillae and taste buds), **Muscles** (voluntary cross-striated muscular fibers), and **Glands** (Mucous Gland, Serous Gland, and Lymph nodes / Tonsils)

Ears

The ear contains sense organs that serve two quite different functions- **Hearing**, and **Postural equilibrium and coordination of head and eye movements.**

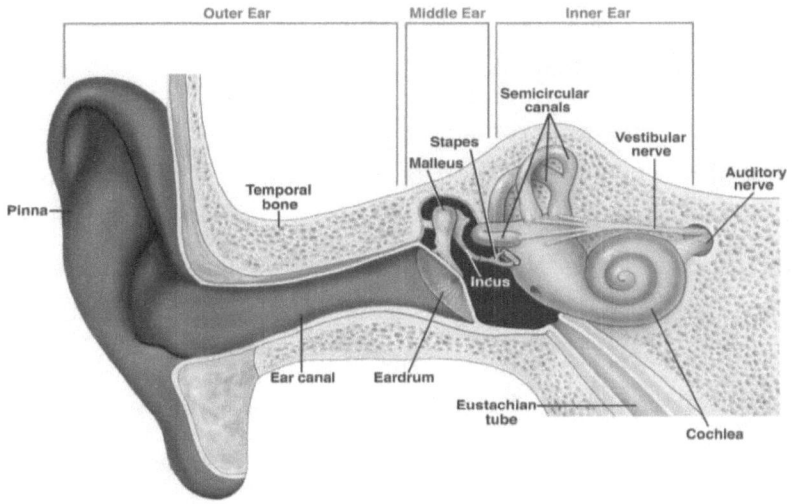

The ear structure can be divided into 3 parts:

Outer Ear- The outer ear is the visible part and is called **the Pinna**. Its job is to collect as many sound waves as possible and channel them into the auditory canal. The sound waves then reach the eardrum. The eardrum is super sensitive to the vibration of air particles (sound waves) so as the air vibrates the eardrum starts to vibrate as well. The eardrum separates the outer ear from the middle ear.

Middle Ear- The middle ear consists of the 3 smallest bones of the body, which together are called ossicles. These are- **The Malleus**/The Hammer, **The Incus**/The Anvil, and **The Stapes**/The Stirrup (This is the shortest among all).

As the eardrum vibrates, the ossicles transfer the sound wave to the inner ear, after amplifying it. Amplification of the sound wave is important because the inner ear is filled with a liquid as opposed to the air in the outer and middle ear and liquid needs more pressure to vibrate. Ossicles increase the pressure by 20x to the original air vibration.

Inner Ear- The inner ear consists of a bony structure. The upper part of this structure consists of 3 semicircular rings which help us in maintaining our balance. The lower part of the ear is a snail-like structure called **Cochlea**. The Cochlea converts the sound wave (air vibration) into electrical impulses. These electrical impulses travel through the auditory nerves all the way to the brain where it gets interpreted as sound.

Hearing and Balance- In the inner ear, there is a ring-like structure called a semicircular canal. These canals are also connected to the Cochlea which is responsible for the sound. These 3 canals are-

- **Superior Semi-circular Canal-** The fluid in these canals moves as the head moves in Yes movements.
- **Posterior Semi-circular Canal-** The fluid here corresponds to the movement when the head tilts down to the shoulder.
- **Lateral Semi-circular Canal-** The fluid here moves when the head moves in a No movement.

Each of these canals contains the fluid called **Endolymph** and hair cells called **Cilia.** Whenever the head moves the fluid moves and so do the cilia. The cilia send signals to the brain about the direction of the head movement. When you sit in a merry-go-round the fluid in these semi- circular canals also starts moving, After some time these fluids start moving at the same rate as you do. Once you stop, the fluid in the canal still keeps moving which sends false information to the brain about the head movement and that's why we feel giddy.

Skin

The skin makes up **16%** of our physical weight. It is the largest organ in the body. If laid down flat it would cover **1.7m2** of the ground. Skin is part of an **integumentary system** (The integumentary system is the set of organs forming the outermost layer of our body) that also includes hair, nail, and exocrine glands such as sweat glands, sebaceous glands, etc.

Skin is made up of 3 layers - **Epidermis, Dermis, and Hypodermis.**

Skin's thickness can vary from **0.5mm at its thinnest up to 4 mm** at its thickest. Three key functions of skin can be categorized as protecting, regulating, and sensing. The skin has many pressure-sensitive components called Merkel cells. In the fingertip alone there are 750 Merkel cells per square cm of skin. These cells are coupled with over 2500 receptors which give us the sense of touch. This surface is also the body's major line of defence against exposure to various foreign elements.

The function of the Skin

- Protection against pathogens. Langerhans cells in the skin are part of the immune system.
- Stores lipid and water, also it is the site of Vitamin D synthesis.
- Nerve endings detect temperature, pressure, vibration, touch, and injury.
- The skin prevents water from escaping by evaporation.

3.3 Homeostasis

Homeo (Similar) + Stasis (a state of stability) (Greek Root)

Homeostasis is the body's ability to maintain a relatively stable internal state that persists despite changes in the world outside. **Physiologist Walter Cannon** coined the term Homeostasis in the 1920s, expanding on the previous work of Physiologist Claude Bernard who coined the term milieu interior.

Homeostasis is maintained at many levels. For instance, the stomach maintains a pH that's different from that of surrounding organs, each individual cell maintains ion concentrations different from those of the surrounding fluid. Apart from these

Homeostasis processes maintain water, oxygen, blood sugar level, and core body temperature.

Function / Mechanism

Maintenance of homeostasis usually involves a **Negative feedback loop**. This is a process where the response itself feeds back negatively (as a new input) to the stimulus to shut down the ongoing process.

These loops act to oppose the stimulus or cue that triggers them. **Such as-** if your body temperature is too high, a negative feedback loop will bring it back down towards the set point of 37 degrees Celsius or 98.6F.

In this case, at first, high temperatures will be detected by sensors. Primarily by the nerve cells with endings in the skin and brain. This information then is relayed to a temperature regulatory control center; Hypothalamus. Hypothalamus will process the information and activate effectors such as the sweat glands, whose job is to oppose the stimulus by bringing body temperature down.

Stimulus---Sensor---Control---Effector---(Repeat)

In the opposite scenario when the body temperature falls in case of cold temperatures, the blood vessels constrict so that heat is conserved. Sweat glands will be inactive and shivering (involuntary contraction of muscles) will be triggered which would generate heat and this would continue until the body achieves normal temperature.

Positive Feedback Loop- This is a process that amplifies the starting signal. Such as the birth of the baby.

3.4 Yogic concept of health and wellness

The qualitative aspect of health is something that yoga and Indian systems of medicine have considered important for thousands of years. The definition of **asana** given in the **Yoga Sutra** as **Sthira Sukham Asanam** implies the state of steady well-being at all levels of existence. Patanjali also tells us that through the practice of **Asana**, we can attain a state that is beyond dualities leading to a calm and serene state of well-being.

- The **World Health Organization (WHO)** defines health as "a state of complete physical, mental, and social well-being". It also states that health is not just the absence of disease or infirmity. However, Yoga understands health and well-being as a dynamic continuum of human nature and not a **mere** state to be attained and maintained.
- Yoga considers that we are not just the physical body but are of a **multifold universal nature**.
- Concepts of **Panchkosh** and **Tri-Sharia /Triguna** help us understand our multidimensional real nature.
- Yoga and Ayurveda consider that the human body is made up of 7 substances **(Sapta Dhatu)- Rasa, Rakta, Mamsa, Meda, Asthi, Majja,** and **Shukra.**
- Both these ancient health sciences understand the importance of tri dosha whose balance is vital for good health.
- Health is further also understood as the harmony of **Pranavayu, Up-prana vayu,** and **stability of nadi with the proper functioning of all chakra.**
- Hatha Yoga Pradipika mentions a state of perfect health and wellness that can be achieved through practicing Hatha Yoga. Swatmaram says that "Perfection of Hatha yoga is achieved

when there is leanness of the body, tranquil countenance, manifestation of the inner sound, clear eyes, disease-lessness, control of Bindu, active digestive fire, and purification of nadis."
- In Patanjali Yoga Sutra, a description of bodily perfection (**Kaya Sampat**) is referred as- "Perfection of the body includes, the beauty of form, grace, strength or energy, and the qualities of power and illuminance of a diamond."

Qualities of mental health according to Yoga-

The quality of a mentally healthy person (**SthitPragya**) is discussed in great detail in **Bhagavad-Gita.** Krishna explains that-

- One whose mind remains undisturbed amidst misery, who does not crave pleasure, and who is free from attachment, fear, and anger, is called a sage of steady wisdom."
- A mentally healthy person is devoid of attachment to possessions, egoism, equipoised in pleasure and distress, and forgiving.
- He / She is firm in understanding and unbewildered.

Maharshi Patanjali emphasis on the simple practice of contentment to achieve the optimum levels of mental health. He tells us that we can gain unexcelled happiness, mental comfort, joy, and satisfaction by practicing contentment.

Importance of psychosocial environment for health and wellness

Psycho-Social environment refers to our interaction with our surroundings and its effect on our mental health. Family, friends, work, society, etc all of these come under our psycho-social environment. Simply put, the kind of people we surround ourselves with, play a very significant role in our overall well-being.

Being subjected to criticism, jealousy, peer pressure, wishing to be likable all the time, wishing to be on the top all the time, financial pressure, etc, are measure that causes worsening mental health. Since we are social animals, we have to learn to conduct ourselves in society, and in order to build strong mental grounds and values, Patanjali has made **Yamas** a mandatory practice.

The practice of **Chitta Prasadana** is another practical technique for ensuring a healthy psycho-social environment.

3.5 Concept of Tridoshas, Sapta Dhatu, Agni, Vayu, and Mala; their role in wellness.

The Tridhosha

The Tridhosha theory is a derivation of the Pancabhautic principle and it forms the foundation of Ayurveda. It has been postulated that whatever physiological and pathological processes occur in the body, they are under the influence of three basic biological elements or humorous known as **Vata, Pitta, and Kapha.**

- Tridhoshas are responsible for maintaining the functional entity of man.
- Trishoshas maintain the body when they are normal & balanced and if there is imbalance and abnormality, the individual becomes diseased.

Vata-

- The term Vata literally means air or wind. It is derived from the root 'Vaa' which denotes movement. Many of the properties of the Vata Dosha are similar to that of the wind. Hence the Dosha is named after it.
- Vata is the most powerful and active Dosha. This is due to its mobility. Other Doshas do not move about actively. They are transported by Vata. Hence Vata is considered the leader of other Dosha.
- Vata is made of all five elements. But **Vayu and Akasha** are very predominant in the combination.
- When increased Vata exhibits signs such as leanness, dark pigmentation, tremor, constipation, weakness, etc.
- When decreased Vata exhibits signs such as a lack of interest in speech, loss of sensation, weakness of the body, etc.

Types of Vata

Vata is divided into five types according to physiology. They are: -

- <u>**Prana (especially moving Vata)**</u> - **Prana** is based in the head and travels from there to the chest through the throat. It regulates and supports intelligence, heart, sense faculties, and mind.
- <u>**Udana (upward Vata)**</u> - **Udana** is based in the chest and travels from there upward to the nose and down to the navel (umbilicus). It is responsible for phonation, effort, energy, strength, complexion, and memory. It is responsible for deep or active respiration. Effort (prayatna) here refers to the stimulation for the initiation of physical activity.

- **Vyana (pervasive Vata)** - **Vyana** is based on the heart and travels throughout the body at high speed. It is responsible for all voluntary movements and many involuntary movements such as the heartbeat. We may say that most of the physical movements are affected by Vyana. It is responsible for the circulation of blood and other body fluids.
- **Samana (equally moving Vata)** - **Samana** is based near the digestive fire in the digestive tract and it travels throughout the gastrointestinal tract. It is responsible for the following-
  - Receipt (Ingestion) of food by the G.I tract (Anna-Grahana),
  - Digestion (Pachana),
  - Separation (Vivechana) of the digested food into essence from undigested,
  - Debris and the release (Mochana) of the debris as feces.
- **Apana (Downward Vata)** - **Apana** is based in the anal canal and travels throughout the pelvis, urinary bladder external genitalia, and thigh. It is responsible for the expulsion of urine and feces, ejaculation, menstruation, and labor.

Pitta-

- The term Pitta is derived from the Sanskrit root 'Tap' which means to heat.
- Pitta is the only Dosha hot in nature. It is analogous to fire. The similarity of Pitta with fire is very much so that it is identified as a product of fire or even as identical to fire.
- Pitta is made of all five elements. But the **Agni & Water** is predominant in the combination.

- When abnormally increased Pitta will impart yellow coloration to feces, urine, eyes, and skin. It will cause excessive thirst and hunger. It will cause insomnia.
- When Pitta is abnormally decreased the digestive power will be reduced. All metabolic activities will become slow and reduced. Then the body becomes cold and lusterless.

Types of Pitta

Name	Location	Function
Pachaka Pitta	Small Intestine	Digestion
Ranjaka Pitta	Liver	Colouring of the blood
Saadhaka Pitta	Heart	Emotional & Mental activities
Aalochaka Pitta	Eye	Vision
Bharajaka Pitta	Skin	Skin Color

Kapha-

- The term Kapha is related to Apas which means water. It indicates that Kapha is basically the product of water.
- Kapha is the builder of the body. It is anabolic in nature and stands for the conservation of energy. It is gross and stable and all the structural material of the living body is the product of Kapha.
- It is responsible for the growth, repair, and nutrition of the body.
- Kapha is predominant in **Bhoomi and Jala** elements.

- When increased Kapha exhibits signs such as a decrease of digestive power, excessive salivation, laziness, feeling of heaviness of the body and undue increase of weight, cough, excessive sleep, etc.
- When decreased Kapha exhibits signs such as dizziness, palpitation, looseness of joints, etc.

Types of Kapha-

Name	Location	Function
Avalambaka Kapha	Heart	Support
Kledaka Kapha	Kledaka Kapha	Lubricate the food
Bodhaka Kapha	Tongue	Taste
Tarpaka Kapha	Eye	Nourishing
Sleshmaka kapha	Joints	Binding

Doshas and the Ayurvedic Clock-

As per Ayurveda, each day is divided into 4-hours dayparts. Each of these dayparts is connected to the slow rise, peaking, and then falling of a particular dosha in our body

Vata time: 2 AM – 6 AM and 2 PM – 6 PM-

During Vata time, we're creative and inquisitive and attuned to the more subtle energies present in the Universe and within ourselves. The morning hours are best for our spiritual practices and inner focus, and the afternoon is best to work and socialize. Both periods are ideal for creative expression.

Kapha time: 6 AM – 10 AM and 6 PM – 10 PM

During Kapha time, our **digestive fire is slower** and our minds are in a restful state. In the morning, we should decrease kapha's sluggishness by being awake, exercising, and eating foods that are stimulating yet easy to digest. In the evening, we should allow our bodies to wind down through a light, nourishing meal, gentle exercise, and self-care.

Pitta time: 10 AM – 2 PM and 10 PM – 2 AM

During Pitta time, our **digestive fire is at its peak**, in terms of both our ability to digest foods and to digest emotions and experiences. The midday period is when we should eat our largest meal of the day, and ideally, we will be sleeping before the nighttime period begins so that we can properly digest and assimilate everything from the day.

Dosha and Season-

Vata:

- This dosha **accumulates** during the dry/ dehydrating heat of the **Summer (Grishma Ritu)**.
- **The rainy season (Varsha Ritu)** makes it **aggravated** which causes indigestion, an acidic atmosphere & gas. In this season, the dryness of the climate is associated with coldness. Both qualities of nature are similar to qualities of Vata and hence favorable to cause its aggravation.
- **Auto-pacification** of Vata takes place in the **Autumn (Sharad Ritu)** season. The excess of heat and oil in the atmosphere is the opposite of Vata, hence Vata gets auto-pacified, provided one follows the seasonal regime.

Pitta:

- This dosha **accumulates** during the **rainy season (Varsha Ritu)** due to the prevailing sourness in the vegetation as a result of excessive rain.
- **Autumn (Sharad Ritu)** makes it **aggravated** when heat returns after the cooling spell of the rainy season. The qualities of excess heat and oil in the atmosphere are similar to Pitta, hence favorable for pitta aggravation.
- **Auto-pacification** of Pitta takes place in the next season - **early winter (Hemant Ritu).** The prevailing coldness and dryness in the atmosphere are the opposite qualities of Pitta. That's why Pitta gets auto-pacified in this season, provided one follows the seasonal regime.

Kapha:

- This dosha **accumulates** during the **cold season (Shishir Ritu)** due to winds, clouds & rain-generated coolness. Excessive coldness causes consolidation of Kapha and hence its accumulation.
- **Spring (Vasant Ritu)** makes it **aggravated** when warm weather liquefies the accumulated Kapha and enables it to flow through the entire body.
- **Auto-pacification** of Kapha takes place in the next season; **Summer (Grishma Ritu).** The excessive heat and dryness of the weather being the opposite qualities of kapha will cause auto-pacification, provided the seasonal regime is being followed.

Dhatu-

- The term Dhatu is roughly correlated with tissue. They are the basic building structures of the living body.
- This term is derived from the Sanskrit root "**dhra**" which means to support. Thus Dhatus are supporting the living body. In other words, they constitute the bulk of the living body.
- **If we remove any of the Dhatu, the body can no more exist as a working mechanism**. That is why the Dhatus are considered supporters of the living body.
- According to Ayurveda, there are seven Dhatus. It is **improper** to strictly correlate them with the tissues according to modern anatomy. Yet for ease of understanding a rough correlation is given below. The correlation is made from the literal meanings of the terms.

Dhatu	Correlated Modern Anatomical Structure
Rasa	Body Fluid
Rakta	Blood
Mamsa	Flesh
Meda	Fat
Asthi	Bone
Majja	Bone-marrow
Shukra	Semen / Ova

Agni-

- Ayurveda considers that digestion and metabolism have a very important role in health and disease. If the biological

transformations in a living system are intact the organism enjoys health.
- If any one or more of such transformations go, wrong disease is the result.
- For each biochemical transformation, there should be a specific transforming agent or Agni.
- Though many scholars, even **Sushruta** consider **Pitta and Agni** to be identical, however from the theoretical point of view they don't look the same.
- **Pitta is categorized as a Dosha whereas the Agni is not considered a Dosha.** Agni works under the control of the three Doshas. Hence it is subordinate to Doshas.
- There are 13 types of Agni.
    - **One Jatharagni (Digestive / Gastric Fire),**
    - **5 Bhootagni (Elemental Fire), and**
    - **7 Dhatvagni (Tissue Fire).**
- Of all the fires the **gastric fire** is the most important as the well-being of all the fires is directly or indirectly related to the normalcy of this fire. Proper digestion is conducive to proper metabolism as the absorbed end products of digestion are the basis for metabolism. If the digestion is not normal, its end products also will be abnormal.

Mala-

- Mala refers to the waste product of the body.
- These are collectively referred to as **Trimala- Stool (Pureesha), Urine (Mootra), and Sweat (Sveda).**

- An increase in **Stool (Pureesha)** will cause heaviness, gurgling sounds, pain, or distention of the abdomen. A decrease in Pureesha will cause the intestines to be filled with gases.
- An increase in **Urine (Mootra)** will cause pricking pain in the bladder or sometimes a feeling that urine is not voided even after voiding it. A decrease in **Urine (Mootra)** will cause a reduction in the output of urine, painful urination, discoloration, or even blood in the urine.
- An increase in **Sweat (Sveda)** will cause excessive sweating, an offensive odor of the body, and Itching of the skin. A decrease in **Sweat (Sveda)** will cause falling or raising of body hair, and cracking of the skin.

3.6 Dinacharya and Ritucharya

Dina Charya-

Dina – Daily Charya – Discipline

Ayurveda advocates daily regimens to be followed by healthy individuals to prevent diseases and maintain health. **Activities done by a person from morning to evening are referred to as Dinacharya.**

It is important to understand that Ayurveda focuses more on the **prevention** of diseases than treatment and Dinacharya is considered a measure to prevent physical, mental, and social problems. Amongst many other factors, Time has been given significant importance in Ayurveda. There are various changes that occur in the body by the impact of time and later on result in the manifestation of various diseases.

If these changes are terminated/controlled by different activities described under Dinacharya, diseases can be prevented. **An ideal Dinacharya includes the following activities-**

Jagran- Waking Up

To maintain health ideal wake-up time is before sunrise i.e., **Brahma Muhoorta**. A Muhoorta is a period of 48 minutes. The day (24 hours) is divided into 30 Muhoorta. The penultimate Muhoorta of the night is named after Brahma, the creator. It begins 96 minutes before sunrise. For instance, when the sunrise is at 06.00 hrs, the time for rousing is from 04.24 hrs to 05.12 hrs. This timing is applicable only when days and nights are equal. When days are longer or shorter, we should make appropriate allowances. Note also that these timings are not meant for the sick.

Vicharana- Contemplation of health

Once awake, before leaving bed one should think of himself in the context of health. It is customary to think the following before leaving the bed.

What is the time? Where am I? What are my incomes and expenses? Who am I? What is my potency? etc.

Malotsarga- Toilets, **Danta Dhavan-** Brushing the teeth, **Anjana-** Application of collyrium, **Nasya-** Nasal instillation of medicine

Gandoosha- Gargle / Oil Pulling - After Nasya, gargling with oil (sesame oil primarily) strengthens the teeth and the muscles of the cheek.

Dhooma Pana- Smoke Inhalation- Inhalation of medicinal smoke clears the throat and upper respiratory channels.

Tamboola Sevana- Chewing of betel leaves - Chewing betel leaves clarifies the mouth and removes the bad smell of breath.

Abhyanga - Application of oil- After the above procedures, the person should apply sesame oil to the body, especially on the scalp, ears, and soles. It cures and prevents diseases due to Vata, prevents wrinkling of the skin, cures fatigue, provides a good texture of the skin, and increases the tone of muscles.

Vyayama- Physical exercises

Mardana- Massage- After exercise, a soft massage may be done. Here self- message will suffice. But if masseurs are available, their services can be utilized.

Udvartana- Powder massage- Instead of mardana, powder massage can also be done.

Snana- Bath

Prasadhana- Cosmetics and Dressing up After the bath, we may use pleasant and harmless cosmetics and dress up properly.

Anna- Food, **Karma-** Profession

Ritu Charya-

Ritu– Seasonal, Charya – Discipline

There are six seasons according to the Ayurvedic classics. This is according to **the climatic conditions of the Indian subcontinent**. However, the basic ideas proposed in the teachings are applicable universally. The lifestyle of human beings is to be tuned to the season to prevent diseases. Hence ayurveda advocates seasonal regimens.

The six seasons (Ritu) in India

Late (second part of) winter - Mid-January to Mid-March – **Shishira**

Spring - Mid-March to Mid-May- **Vasanta**

Summer - Mid-May to Mid-July- **Greeshma**

Rainy season - Mid-July to Mid-September- **Varsha**

Autumn - Mid-September to Mid-November- **Sharad**

Early (first part of) winter- Mid-November to Mid-January- **Hemanta**

Solstices

The first three seasons together constitute the **northern solstice**. It is a debilitating period as the Sun extracts energy and is called the 'taking time.' **The latter three seasons** constitute the **southern solstice**. It is the 'giving time' when nature gives energy to living beings. It is the strengthening period.

Name of the months in Hindi-

Chaitra (March-April), **Vaishakha** (April-May), **Jyestha** (May-June), **Ashadha** (June-July), **Shravan** (July- Aug), **Bhadrapada** (Aug-Sep), **Ashvin** (Sep-Oct), **Kartika** (Oct- Nov), **Aghana/ Marga-Sheersha** (Nov- Dec), **Pausha** (Dec-Jan), **Magha** (Jan-Feb), **Falguna** (Feb-March)

Seasons and Strength-

Maximal strength – in winter, **Medium strength** - in spring & autumn **Minimal strength** – in rainy & summer

Seasons and Taste-

Of the six tastes, one taste becomes prominent in each season. The predominant tastes (in vegetables etc.) during the seasons are-

Shishira – bitter, **Vasanta**- astringent, **Greeshma** – pungent, **Varsha** – sour, **Sharad** – salt, **Hemanta** – sweet

Junction of seasons-

When a season ends and another season sets in there will be an intermediate period of the **junction of seasons.** During this period practices of the outgoing season are to be **tapered off** and practices of the incoming season are to be gradually assumed. The change of practice should not be abrupt.

3.7 Importance of Ahara, Nidra, and Brahmacharya in well-being-

3 Pillars Of Health - Trayopstambha

An optimal state of Health, or 'Svastha', according to Ayurveda, can only be achieved when there is a proper balance of the **"Three Pillars of Life."** These pillars are so revered in the tradition that the Charaka Samhita says that, "one who manages these three pillars properly is guaranteed a full life span that will not be cut short by disease." Every Ayurveda treatment protocol brings attention to restoring balance within these three areas. The 'Trayopastambha' or Three Pillars of Health are:

- **Right Diet - Ahara**
- **Right Sleep - Nidra**
- **Right Sexuality - Brahmacharya**

These are an essential and integral part of our lives, and when they find harmony, the body, mind, and heart follow in living to their full potential.

Right Diet (Ahara)-

- Proper diet, digestion, and elimination are paramount to our well-being.
- Through proper digestion, our bodies are able to absorb from the food all the nutrients and the vital life-force energy **(Prana)** that acts as the building blocks of our bodies and minds.
- Proper digestion, according to Ayurveda, has various levels. The ultimate gift of proper digestion is **Ojas**, our subtle vital energy that protects the body and mind from disease and gives us great vigor and longevity.
- Proper digestion requires the intake of the ideal foods for a person's constitution. It also requires that food be consumed properly, with mindfulness, at proper timings, and in proper combination.
- When the choice of food is not appropriate for the constitution of the person or the food is taken improperly, the result is a disturbance of one or more of the body's three doshas (Vata, Pitta, or Kapha).
- Improper digestion eventually results in disease.

- Easeful, balanced digestion for all doshic types should bring lightness, joy, and peace of body and mind.

Right Sleep (Nidra)-

- Proper rest is essential for the well-being of any person.
- The body utilizes sleep as an opportunity to use its energy for healing and repairing damage to the body that accumulated during waking hours.
- If the body does not receive enough sleep, the body cannot repair the damage caused by stress and strain. This leads to the body breaking down.
- Too much or too little sleep brings on consequences. Too little sleep upsets Vata dosha, while too much disturbs Kapha dosha. Disturbance of Vata dosha results in weaker tissues that are more susceptible to injury.
- Disturbance of Kapha dosha results in tissues that become excessive, stagnant, lethargic, and immobile.
- As per Ayurveda, it is important to work with the body clock in order to maintain the sleep-wake cycle. That means, sleeping during the night hours and waking up in Brahma Muhurta.

Right Sexuality (Brahmacharya)-

- Sexuality and its indulgence can become an area of imbalance when engaged excessively and/or 'inappropriately'. Like every activity in our lives, the way we engage in action is as impactful as the action itself (think about mindful eating).
- Ayurveda promotes bringing a quality of Sattva (purity) into everything we do to allow for balance, ease, and lightness at every level of our being - body, mind, and consciousness.

- Excessive or solely pleasure-seeking, lustful sexual activity can be depleting to vital reserves and is contraindicated for those suffering from any disease.

3.8 Knowledge of common diseases;

Their prevention and management by Yoga.

Disease, Disorder, Syndrome, and Condition

Disease- A Disease is defined as a result of the pathological response of the body to either external or internal factors. It is also referred to as abnormalities that can cause physical or emotional stress and pain. The treatment of disease is based on such abnormalities.

Disorder- A Disorder is believed to be the disruption of the usual bodily functions. It is caused because of the presence of disease in the body.

Syndrome vs. Disease- Syndromes are groups of symptoms associated with a disease. Knowing the syndrome can help diagnose the disease.

Condition- A condition indicates your state of health. It is an abnormal state that feels different from your normal state of well-being. Often, you'll hear about someone's condition when they are hospitalized and noted as being in stable or critical condition.

Acidity- (Psychosomatic Disorders)

Physiology- The sphincter muscle acts as a closing between the stomach and the esophagus. It closes as soon as the food passes through the food pipe and into the stomach. In case the sphincter muscle is not able to close properly or if it closes and opens again, the acid from the stomach can move into the esophagus. This condition is referred to as acid reflux. The term acidity is often used to refer to the condition of acid reflux. Frequent episodes of acid reflux could also indicate a case of **GERD (Gastro-esophageal Reflux Disease).**

Symptoms- Heartburn, Bitter taste in the mouth, Headache, Nausea, Burping

Possible Causes- Alcoholism, Smoking, A high intake of table salt, A diet low in dietary fiber, Lying down immediately after eating a meal, and Stress.

Yoga as management and prevention-

As per a study published in the **International Journal of Yog** in July 2013, they found **Agnisar Kriya** and **Kapalbhati** to be particularly useful in addressing acid reflux and GERD, as they can increase diaphragmatic tone. Thus decreasing reflux from the stomach to the esophagus. As per the same study, yoga may also be beneficial in alleviating GERD by impacting the Autonomous Nervous System which limits the ability of the GI tract to continue peristaltic contractions and prevents appropriate fluid and secretion shifts needed for digestion.

Start taking a look at dietary habits. Just by controlling the diet, one can see a lot of difference in Acid reflux. Drink lukewarm water immediately after waking up.

It has been seen that people with acid reflux feel difficulty in lying straight on the back. Keeping the upper back a little elevated while sleeping might help.

Note: The Yoga practice should be done **first thing** in the morning on an empty stomach.

Asana- Mandukasana, Yoga Mudrasana, Bhujangasana, Dhanurasana

Pranayama- Shunyak Pranayama (Bahya Kumbhaka), Yogic breath, Nadi Shodhan

Kriya- Vaman Dhauti, Agnisar Kriya

Constipation

Physiology- Constipation occurs when bowel movements become less frequent and stool becomes difficult to pass. This happens because your colon absorbs too much water from the stool, which dries out the stool and makes it hard in consistency and difficult to push out of the body.

Possible Causes- Low fiber diet, Dehydration, not enough physical movement, Eating large amounts of milk or cheese, Changes in regular routines., Resisting the urge to have a bowel movement, Stress.

Yoga as Management and Prevention - Build awareness about the daily routine, after getting up focus on the "Shaucha" (Toilet). Don't develop habits of taking mobile/newspapers in the toilet. Drink lukewarm water immediately after waking up. Increase fibers in the diet. Practice sitting in Vajrasana for 5-10 mins after every meal.

Note: The Yoga practice should be done first thing in the morning on an empty stomach.

Kriya- Agnisara Kriya, Vaman Dhauti, Laghu Shankha Prakshalana (only once, at the beginning of the program)

Asana- Sukshma Vyayama- Udar Shakti Vikasaka, Pawanmuktasana Part 2 (Abdominal group), Surya Namaskar, Mandukasana, Yoga Mudrasana, Paschimottasana, Vajrasana, Bhujangasana, Dhanurasana, Shalabhasana

Pranayama – Sectional Breathing, Yogic deep breathing, Nadi Shodhan

IBS (irritable bowel syndrome)

Physiology- IBS is one of the major gastrointestinal disorders. It can cause bouts of stomach cramps, bloating, diarrhea, and constipation. In this condition, the partially digested food either moves too quickly or too slowly in the colon. **In the former case**, the colon doesn't have enough time to absorb the water, and this results in diarrhea bouts.

In the latter case, the colon absorbs too much water hence the stool becomes very hard to pass, which results in constipation. Depending upon the above two reactions of the colon, IBS can be classified into two types- **Diarrhoea Predominant, and Constipation Predominant.**

Possible Causes- Stress, unhealthy eating habits, Lack of physical activity.

Yoga as management and prevention- Same as Constipation.

Bronchial Asthma

Physiology- This is also called **"Inflammatory Response Disease"** as the body overreacts to specific environmental agents. In this condition, the airway path of the lungs gets swollen and becomes narrow. Due to this swelling, the air path produces excess mucus making it hard to breathe which results in coughing, short breath, and wheezing. In this disease, "exhaling" becomes more difficult than inhaling, which may result in having more air in the lungs and affects oxygen circulation in the body. This may result in death.

Possible Causes- Genetic, Environmental

Yoga as Management and Prevention-

Learning to exhale efficiently is more important.

Burn a candle and blow it. Practice this a couple of times.

Take a glass of water and blow air through the straw. Watch the bubbles, if the bubbles are coming with obstruction, then it shows your breath is obstructed.

Kriya- Kapalbhati (Should be done very slowly), Simha Kriya

Pranayama –Shunyak/Bahya Kumbhaka (External Retention), Bhramari, Bhastrika (Should be done very slowly)

Asana-Tadasana, Padahastasana, Paschimottasana, Yoga-Mudrasana, Ushtrasana, Dhanurasana, Bhujangasana, Marjaryasana, Bitilasana, Meru Vakrasana

Sinusitis

Physiology-This is an inflammation of the **paranasal sinuses**. The sinuses are small, air-filled cavities behind the cheekbones. There are 4 pairs of sinuses, behind the forehead, on either side of the bridge of the nose, and behind the eyes. The sinuses open up into the cavity of the nose and help control the temperature and water content of the air reaching into the lungs. The mucus produced naturally by the sinuses usually drains into the nose through small channels. These channels can become blocked when the sinuses are infected and inflamed.

Possible Causes- Allergies, Respiratory Tract Infection, Nasal Polyps (A tissue growth that can block the nasal passages or sinuses).

Yoga as management and prevention-

Steam inhalation is very effective in opening the blocked sinus.

Kriya- Jalneti, Sutraneti, Tratak, Kapalbhati, Simha Kriya

Pranayama- Bhastrika, Nadi Shodhan, Ujjayi, Bhramri

Asana- Trikonasana, Konasana, Tadasana, Hastottanasana, Matsyasana, Bhujangasana, Simhasana, Dhanurasana,

Hypertension

Physiology- This is a condition when the force of the blood on the wall of the arteries is often too high. In the heart, two chambers called ventricles contract with each heartbeat to push blood to the lungs and through the arteries to the body. As the blood flows through them, **three main factors** affect the pressure in the artery wall-

Cardiac Output- This is the amount of blood ventricles pushed out of the heart each minute, The BP goes up as the cardiac output increases.

Blood Volume- This refers to the total blood volume in the body. The BP also goes up as the blood volume increases.

Resistance- Anything working against the blood flow through the artery is resistance. A few factors that contribute to resistance are- the flexibility of the artery wall, Artery Diameter, Blood Viscosity / Thickness.

Symptoms- Persistent Headache, Blurred or double vision, Nose bleeds, Shortness of breath.

HBP can be categorized under 2 categories- **Primary Hypertension-** High Bp in the absence of any underlying disease, and **Secondary Hypertension-** Elevated BP due to some underlying disease.

Possible Causes- Stress, Age, Obesity, Excess salt intake, Tobacco, Not being physically active.

Yoga as Management and Prevention-

Kriya- Jalneti, Sutra Neti

Asana- Pawanmuktasana Part 1 and 2, Tadasana, Kati-Chakrasana, Hastottanasana, Vajrasana, Ushtrasana, Gomukhasana, Shashankasana, Vakrasana, Bhujangasana, Makarasana, Shavasana

Pranayama- Nadi Shodhan (Without Retention), Bhramari, Ujjayi, Sheetali,

Meditation- Breath Awareness, Om Chanting

Contraindication- The headstand (topsy-turvy) postures and hyperventilation breathing practices such as Kapalbhati, Bhastrika, etc. should be avoided.

Neck Pain

Physiology- Neck pain is a common complaint. Neck muscles can be strained from poor posture, whether it's leaning over your computer or hunching over your workbench, or scrolling through social media on your phone.

Possible Causes- Muscle Strain, Wear and tear in the joint, Nerve compression, Injuries

Yoga as management and prevention-

Neck Sukshma Vyayama, take 5-10 mins of break and do the light neck stretches every 2 hours of sitting.

Cervical Spondylosis

Physiology- Cervical Spondylosis is a general term for age/posture- related wear and tear affecting the spinal disc in the neck (C1-C7). Usually, the site of the injury is the neck but the pain radiates from one of the shoulders down towards the elbow. Cervical pain is not a constant pain, instead, it gets generated through some triggers such as sudden jerk in the neck. Normally Pain goes away after a few days of rest and rehabilitation. **If the trigger can be understood then preventing cervical gets much easier.**

Possible Causes- Dehydrated Disk, Herniated Disk, Stiff Ligaments

Yoga as management and prevention-

Neck Sukshma Vyayama except chin down movement, Shoulder Sukshma Vyayama, Trikonasana, Bhujangasana (all variations), Ushtrasana, Dhanurasana, Shalabhasana

Contraindication-Vipareeta Karani, Sarvangasana, Setu-bandh asana, Halasana, Chin locking, Jalandhara Bandha, Ujjayi

Lower Back Ache

Physiology- Most people may experience low back pain at a certain stage in their life. It is characterized by pain, stiffness, and tension in the back. This pain can vary from mild to severe depending on duration. It can be short-lived or long-lasting. However, low back pain can make the everyday activity difficult to perform.

Possible Causes- Incorrect sitting, driving or bending posture, lifting, carrying, pushing, or pulling heavy weights incorrectly, sudden jerks, sports injuries

Yoga as management and prevention-

Asana- Lying Spinal Twist (All Variations), Setu Bandhasana, Bhujangasana, Dhanurasana, Shalabhasana

Contraindication- Forward Bending movements.

Arthritis

Physiology- Arthritis is a common condition, characterized by pain and inflammation in the joints, this is due to a number of factors like genetic predisposition, inflammation, altered immune response, metabolic changes, and others. All forms of joint diseases can be best understood in terms of the following pathological process-

Degenerative Joint Disease- Osteoarthritis (OA), Cervical Spondylosis.

Auto Immune Joint Disease- Rheumatoid Arthritis (RA), Psoriatic Arthritis, Lupus.

Metabolic Joint Disease- Gouty Arthritis (GA)

Common Types of Arthritis Disease

Osteoarthritis-

It is a degenerative joint disease in which the cartilage that covers the ends of bones in the joint deteriorates, causing pain and loss of movement as bones begin to rub each other. It is the most common form of arthritis.

Yoga as Management and Prevention- Pawanmuktasana 1, 2 and 3

Contraindication- The hyperflexion or excessive bending of the affected joint is to be avoided completely. Attention should be paid to strengthening the surrounding muscles of the affected joint. Such as in the case of knee arthritis, thigh, and calf strengthing should also be done.

Rheumatoid Arthritis- It is an **autoimmune disease** in which the joint linings get inflamed as a result of abnormal immune response of the body. Rheumatoid arthritis is one of the most serious and disabling types, affecting mostly women.

Yoga as management, prevention, and contraindication- Same as Above

Gout (Gouty Arthritis)- It affects mostly men. It happens due to metabolic disturbance in which increased **uric acid** settles down in the joint spaces causing inflammation. This painful condition most often attacks small joints, especially the big toe.

Yoga as management, prevention, and contraindication- Same as Above. Toe, and finger movements should definitely be included in particular.

Knowledge of the role of Yoga in the management of Metabolic Disorder and Non-Communicable Diseases -

Metabolism- This is the process by which the body converts whatever we eat and drink into energy.

Metabolic Disorder- A metabolic disorder occurs when abnormal chemical reactions in the body disrupt the above-mentioned process. When this happens, the body makes too much or too little of some substances. Metabolic syndrome is not an illness in itself. Rather, it's a gathering of dangerous elements - **hypertension, high glucose, higher cholesterol levels, and stomach fat.**

Examples of metabolic disorders- **PCOS, Type 2 diabetes, etc.**

Yoga as Management and Prevention- Yoga practices are ideal to manage as well as control metabolic disorders in combination with healthy eating habits and lifestyle changes.

The disease-specific program should focus on stimulating the affected organ or the process. Such as for **Menstrual Disorders** asana which stretches and strengthens the **pelvis girdle** such as Malasana, Kashtha Takshanasana, Vayu Nishkasana, etc. should be included.

For **Diabetes management**, the target organ is the pancreas which is a deep-rooted organ. All the asana which creates a deep twist in the spine is ideal here such as- Vakrasana. Ardha-Matsyendrasana, Bhu- Namanasnaa, Parivritta Janu Sheershasana, etc.

Non-communicable Diseases (NCDs)-

NCDs refer to a group of conditions that are not spread through infection to other people, but are caused mainly by prolonged unhealthy behaviours. NCDs usually require long-term treatment and care. **The most common 4 NCDs are- Cardiovascular Disease, Diabetes, Cancer, and Chronic Lung Disorder.**

Yoga as Management

As a general rule physical Activity is crucial to manage NCDs. Yogic practices can be an excellent tool to complement medical treatment and improve overall well-being and quality of life.

Concept of stress and Yogic management of stress

Stress- Stress is the body's reaction to a challenge or demand. Stress is a feeling of emotional or physical tension. It can come from any event or thought that makes you feel frustrated, angry, or nervous. As per Dr. Selye and Levi, "**The primary function of stress is to prepare the body for physical activity such as resistance or flight**. If however, the subject lacks the means of restoring either to fight or flight i.e. of relieving the stress reaction, **stress gives rise to distress** which manifests itself in the form of psychosomatic symptoms or disorders.

The factors of 21st-century stress

- A 24*7 society where everything and everyone is accessible all the time. The downside of this is **poor boundaries**. Poor boundaries tend to be **violated** hence making one feel **victimized**.
- What's interesting is that boundaries are not always violated by others. Most of the time it's **Us Vs Us**. Such as poor boundaries between technology and privacy, between credit and debit, with television, internet, food, etc.
- The rapid rate of change, from technology to economics to family dynamics
- The growing threat of terrorism, global warming, and other changing world dynamics.
- Greater responsibilities, peer pressure, pressure to be in a certain way on social media, and because of that seemingly less freedom.

As the saying goes: Once a victim, twice a volunteer. It is strongly suggested to learn from your experiences and strengthen your personal boundaries as needed so you don't fall prey to **"victim consciousness."**

Nature Of Stress- Stress could be of two natures- **Eustress and Distress.**

Eustress- This is short-term and is produced by joy or any other kind of positive impulse, sensible recreational activities, sports, hobbies, etc. Such as Receiving a promotion or raise at work, starting a new job, having a child, getting married, buying a home, holiday, etc.

Distress- This can be short as well as long-term. This needs to be controlled as it causes anxiety or concern and can lead to mental or physical problems. Such as the death of a spouse, filing for divorce, hospitalization, Illness, being abused or neglected, unemployment, financial problems, etc.

Types of Stress- Stress can generally be divided into 3 categories-

Acute Stress, Episodic Acute Stress, and Chronic Stress.

1. **Acute Stress-** Acute stress happens to everyone. It is the body's immediate reaction to a new and challenging situation. It's the kind of stress you might feel when you narrowly escape a car accident. Acute stress can also come out of something that you actually enjoy. It's the somewhat frightening yet thrilling feeling one gets on a roller coaster or when skiing down a steep mountain slope. Once the danger passes, the body's systems should return to normal. Although Severe Acute Stress is a different story. This kind of stress, such as when you've faced a life-threatening situation, can lead to PTSD (Post Traumatic Stress Disorder) or other mental health problems.

2. **Episodic Acute Stress-** This is the state in which one has frequent episodes of acute stress. This might happen if one

is often anxious and worried about things one suspects may happen. Certain professions, such as law enforcement or firefighters might also lead to frequent high-stress situations. As, with severe acute stress, episodic acute stress can affect your physical health and mental well-being.

3. **Chronic Stress-** When one has high-stress levels for an extended period of time, one has chronic stress. Long-term stress like this can have a negative impact on one's health and leads to Anxiety, Cardiovascular Disease, Depression, HBP, etc.

The physiological changes during stress

When someone experiences a stressful event, **"The amygdala"** which is an area of the brain that contributes to emotional processing, sends a distress signal to the **hypothalamus**. The hypothalamus is like a command center that communicates with the rest of the body through the nervous system. Hypothalamus signals the Sympathetic Nervous System to trigger the **Fight or Flight response**.

As a result, the adrenal glands start releasing the **epinephrine (Adrenaline)** and cortisol hormones, the heart starts to pump the blood faster which results in an increased heartbeat, the lungs start to function faster which results in less oxygen utilization, and alternate breathing channels get activated which results in faster and shallow breathing. **Overall body is all set for whatever is to come.**

Understand that choosing either of the responses, **Flight or Fight** should result in ensuring that the stressful event is over. Once the **amygdala** receives the information that the threat is over, the cortisol level starts to drop. and after 15-20 minutes the **Parasympathetic Nervous System** triggers the opposite response called **Rest or Digest / Feed or Breed**. This opposite response brings the body back to **homeostasis.**

This seems simple but what goes wrong?

The problem occurs **when we fail to choose either fight or flight**. That means that the brain is not receiving the signal that the stressful situation is over. That consequently means that all the body preps are still on, heart rate is still high, breathing is still shallow, oxygen is still not getting properly utilized/metabolized, cortisol is still releasing and slowly building up, and the Parasympathetic Nervous system is not getting the signal to trigger the opposite response. **Think of it as you have switched on a motor but forgot to switch it off.**

Also understand that when Cortisol is released in moderation, it helps in restoring balance to the body after a stressful event. It regulates blood sugar levels in cells and has utilitarian value in the Hippocampus, where memories are stored and processed. But in the case of **chronic stress,** the body makes **more cortisol** than it has a chance to release. High levels of cortisol can **wear down** the brain's ability to function properly. Stress can **kill** brain cells and even reduce the **size** of the brain. Cortisol is believed to create a domino effect between the Hippocampus, and Amygdala in a way that might create a vicious cycle by creating a brain that becomes predisposed to be in a constant state of **fight-flight.**

This continuous state of being in stress eventually leads to **permanent consequences** such as the increased risk of heart disease, HBP, Diabetes, Irregular Breathing, Cervical, Shoulder pain, Arthritis, Eating disorders, Depression, Anxiety, and Insomnia. It can even impair the body's immune system.

Doctors agree that almost all diseases can be a manifestation of mental stress, aka, being unable to switch off the motor.

Specific Practices for Stress Management

Asana- Surya Namaskara, Pawanmuktasana Part 3 (Shakti Bandha Group), Asanas in which the spine arches, bends, and twists, All the asanas in which the shoulders are engaged actively

Pranayama- Sectional Breathing, Full Yogic breath, Ujjayi, Bhramri, Nadi Shodhan, Bahya Kumbhaka.

Mental Attitude- Yama and Niyama. Pratipaksha Bhavana, Abhyasa & Vairagya, Karma Yoga, Bhakti Yoga.

Meditation- In the cases of depression, anxiety, overthinking, etc inward practices such as Dhyana, Yoga Nidra, etc. **might not be helpful** as the overthinking pattern of such practitioners might increase if they are left alone with their thoughts for a longer duration. The flow of destructive thoughts will be unconsciously higher in such practitioners.

Instead of the usual meditation practices, **Repeating Affirmations** (if possible, loudly), **Om chanting**, and Mantra Chants such as **Guruashtakam** multiple times in a day work best to keep the willpower strong.

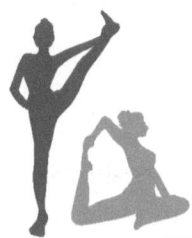

UNIT 4

PRACTICAL

4.1 Prayer:

Concept and Recitation Of Pranava and Hymns, Selected universal prayers, invocations, and Nishpatti Bhava.

Prayer is an indispensable part of our lives, irrespective of culture. The impulse to ask for divine assistance is an integral part of being human. Traditionally, a yoga class always starts and ends with a **Mantra** which is a prayer in Sanskrit. It is necessary to know the proper pronunciation, intonation, and meaning of the chant in order to understand as well as experience the full benefits. Bhagwad Gita also emphasizes **that mechanical chanting** doesn't yield many benefits.

Recitation of Hymns-

Hymns are understood as religious songs in praise or prayer of a particular deity. The word hymn is derived from the Greek word- **hymnos "a song of praise."**

On a physical level, the chanting impacts the parts from where the **chant notes are raised** such as-abdomen, the lungs, the circulatory system, the back of the throat, etc. The rhythmic chanting creates a neuro-linguistic effect, even if the meaning of the mantra is not known.

However, knowing the **meaning** of chanting tunes our mind towards reaching our goal. It is highly suggested to understand the meaning of the mantra and chant with faith. This leads to spiritual awakening as the mind gets focused. Research shows the increased effect of releasing healing chemicals in the brain when we are intentionally attaching a meaning or understanding to the mantra. This is called the **Psycholinguistic effect (PLE).**

Nishpatti Bhava-

Nishpatti bhava is a term used to describe the state of spiritual realization and the ultimate goal of self-discovery and liberation. It represents the realization of one's true nature or the recognition of the underlying unity and oneness of all things.

Selected universal prayers

Gayatri Mantra

Origin- Rigveda, The Rishi of this mantra is **Vishvamitra,** the devata is **Savitr,** the Chhanda is **Gayatri** (one of the metrical forms adopted in Rigveda).

Om- Bhūr- Bhuva- Svah, Tat- Savitur- Varenyam |

Bhargo- Devasya- Dhimahi, Dhiyo- Yo- Nah- Prachodayat ||

Om: The primeval sound, **Bhur:** the physical realm, **Bhuvah:** the mental realm, **Svah:** the spiritual realm, **Tat:** That (God), **Savitur:** the Sun, **Vareñyam:** adore, **Bhargo:** effulgence, **Devasya:** supreme Lord, **Dhīmahi:** meditate, **Dhiyo:** the intellect, **Yo:**

May this light (used as a pronoun referring to the Sun), **Nah:** our, **Prachodayat:** illumine/ inspire.

Meaning- We meditate on that most adored Supreme Lord, Sun, the creator, whose effulgence illuminates all realms (physical, mental, and spiritual). May this divine light illuminate our intellect.

Shanti Mantra

Origin- Mentioned in Puranas, this verse was also musically adapted, particularly for the purpose of service and prayers in **Brahmo temples**, by Rabindranath Tagore.

Om- Sarve- Bhavantu- Sukhinah, Sarve- Santu- Niramayah | Sarve- Bhadraanni- Pashyantu, Maa- Kashcid- Duhkha- Bhaag- Bhavet ||Om Śhāntiḥ, Śhāntiḥ, Śhāntiḥ ||

Om- The primeval sound, **Sarve-** All, **Bhavantu-** To be, **Sukhinah-** Happy or prosperous, **Santu-** To be, **Niraa-** Free, **Aamayaha-** Illness, **Bhadhrani-** Good or auspicious, **Pashyantu-** May see, **Ma-** Not or never, **Kashchit-** Anyone, **Dukha-** Suffering, **Bhag-** Portion, **Bhavet-** Experience,

Meaning- May all be happy; May all be free from infirmities; May all see good; May none partake in suffering. May there be Peace, Peace, Peace.

Pavmana Mantra

Origin- Brihadaranyaka Upanishad, Pavmana means "being purified, strained".

Om Asato Maa Sad-Gamaya, Tamaso Maa Jyotir-Gamaya |

Mrityor-Ma Amritam Gamaya, Om Śhāntiḥ, Śhāntiḥ, Śhāntiḥ ||

Asataḥ- from falsehood, **Ma**- not /Never, **Sat** - to truth, **Gamaya** - lead, **Tamasaḥ** - from darkness, **Jyotiḥ** - to light, **Mṛtyoḥ**- from death, **Amritam**- to immortality

Meaning- From falsehood, lead me to truth, From darkness, lead me to light, From death, lead me to immortality. May there be Peace, Peace, Peace.

Shanti Mantra

Origin- IshaVasya Upanishad. This mantra is commonly chanted as a prayer before the study of the Upanishad begins. This is a mantra of the most significant statements ever made anywhere on earth at any time.

Om Poornam-adah Poornam-idam, Poornat-Poornam-udachyate |

Poorna-asya Poornam-aadaya Poornam-eva-Avashissyate

||Om Shantih, Shantih, Shantih ||

Om - Symbol of Para brahman, **Purnnam-Adah** -That (Adah; referred as a pronoun for outer world) is Purna (Full with Divine Consciousness), **Purnam-Idam**- This (Idam- referred as pronoun for a inner world] is also Purna (Full with Divine Consciousness), **Poornat** - From Fullness, **Poornam** - Fullness, **Udachyate**- To be thrown out, **Poornasya**- Of Fullness, **Poorna**- Fullness, **Aadaya**- Taking, **Poorna**: Fullness, **Eva:** Indeed/Truly, **Avashissyate:** will remain.

Meaning- THAT is infinite, THIS is infinite; From That, THIS comes. THIS added or removed from THAT, the Infinite remains as Infinite. Om, peace, peace, peace.

Patanjali Invocation Mantra

This invocation to Patanjali is the introduction to the **Bhoja Vritti**, the commentary on the Yoga Sutras written by **Raja Bhoj.**

Yogena - chittasya- padena- vācāṁ, Malaṁ - śarīrasya - ca - vaidyakena|

Yo'pākarottaṁ - pravaraṁ - munīnāṁ, Patañjaliṁ - prāñjalirānato'smi||

Ābahu - puruṣākāraṁ Śaṅkha - cakrāsi - dhāriṇaṁ|

Sahasra - śīrasaṁ - śvetaṁ, Pranamāmi - Patañjaliṁ ||

Meaning- Yoga that brings quietness of mind; grammar that elicits effective speech and the healing arts that remove bodily ailments. He is the most illustrious of sages Patanjali to whom I bow down. I bow to Patanjali, who has an upper body like a human, who holds a conch shell (shankha) and a discus (chakra), who has a thousand radiant heads, and who is white in complexion.

4.2 Yogic Shat Karma:

Neti: Sutra Neti and Jala Neti Dhauti: Vamana Dhauti (Kunjal), Kapalbhati (Vatakrama)

Refer to Unit 1.10 for Shatkarma, In the demonstration exam only these 3 karmas will be asked. You have to be prepared with Instructions, 2 benefits, and 2 contraindications.

It is highly suggested to first practice these karmas as part of your preparation under the guidance.

4.3 Yogic Sukshma & Sthula Vyayama

Neck Movement: Griva Shakti Vikasaka (I,II,III)

Technique I - Turn the neck **right and left** repeatedly in a swift motion.

Technique 2 - Bring the chin to the chest then **rotate the neck** from the right shoulder to the left shoulder and reverse. Always do **half-neck rotation** since the neck is a pivot joint.

Technique 3- Inhale while tightening the throat muscles. Exhale and relax.

Shoulder Movement: Bhuja Valli Shakti Vikasaka, Purna Bhuja Shakti Vikasaka

Bhuja Valli Shakti Vikasaka- Stand upright with feet together. Inhale and take the right arm straight up, exhale and drop. Repeat with the other side.

Purna Bhuja Shakti Vikasaka (Arm Rotation)- Stand upright with feet together. Make a fist with both palms and rotate the arms vigorously. Continue breathing.

Trunk Movement: Kati Shakti Vikasaka (I, II, III, IV, V)

Technique I- Stand upright with feet together. Make a fist of the right palm and grab the right wrist by the left palm, keeping the palms behind your back. Inhale and arch your back, exhale and bend forward. Do this in a dynamic fashion.

Technique II- Stand upright with feet wide as much as possible. Keep both palms on the waist with thumbs facing the front and fingers towards the back. Inhale and arch your back and exhaling, bend forward trying to touch the crown on the ground. Do this in a dynamic fashion.

Technique III- Stand upright with feet together. Keep your palms by the side of the body. Inhale and arch your back, exhaling bend forward. Ensure that while doing this movement, arms do not touch the thighs.

Technique IV- Stand upright with feet together. Straighten the arms sideways up to the level of the shoulders. Inhale and exhaling, and bend your body towards the right leg, keeping a straight back.

Inhale, come back to the center and exhale bend to the other side.

Knee Movement: Jangha Shakti Vikasaka (II- A& B), Janu Shakti Vikasaka

Jangha Shakti Vikaska II- A- (Squats) Stand with keeping the feet together. Extend your arms in front of you keeping them parallel to the ground. Now, inhale and exhaling bend from the knees in squatting position, bring the thighs parallel to the ground and knees over the toes, and hold the position for as long as you can.

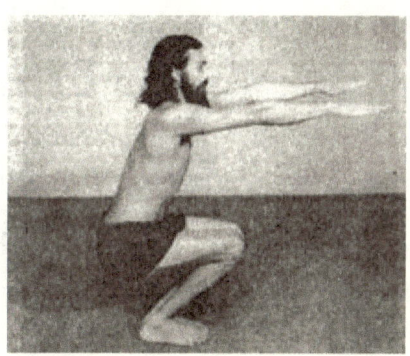

Jangha Shakti Vikaska II- B- (Squats- II) Stand with keeping the toes together and knees apart. Extend your arms sideways like wings.

Now, inhale and exhaling bend from the knees in a manner that knees open to the sideways, maintain the balance on the toes.

Hold the position for as long as you can.

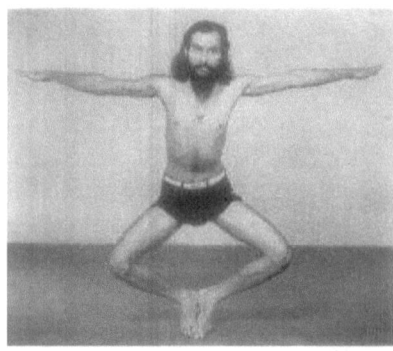

Janu Shakti Vikasaka (Heels to the hips) - Stand upright with feet together. Lift your right leg straight up to 20 inches off the floor and with a jerk touch the heel to the right hip. Again, straighten the leg and place it on the floor. Repeat with the other leg.

Ankle Movement: Pada-Mula-Shakti-Vikasaka (A&B)

Pada-Mula-Shakti-Vikasaka A (Heel and Toe movement)- Stand tall with feet together and arms by the side of the body. Stand on the toes and then on the heels in a swift motion.

Pada-Mula-Shakti-Vikasaka B (Jumping on the toes)- Come on to the toes and jump on the toes continuously.

Gulpha-Pada-Pristha-pada-tala-shakti-Vikasaka (Ankle Rotation)-

Stand tall with feet together and arms by the side of the body. Lift the right leg straight in front of you and rotate the ankle clockwise and then in the anti-clockwise direction. Repeat with the other leg.

Yogic Sthula Vyayama (Macro Circulation Practices)
Sarvanga Pushti-

- Stand tall with feet wide up to 3 feet distance. Raise your arms above your head and interlock the fingers, inhale arch your back turn towards the right leg. Exhaling, bend your upper body towards the right leg.
- Inhale and stand tall. Once again arching your back turn towards the left leg and with the next exhalation bend towards the left leg.
- This whole movement should be done in a swift motion.

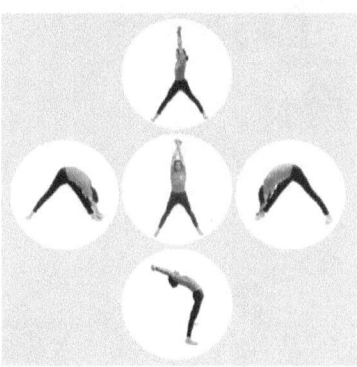

Hrid Gati-

Stand tall with both feet together and arms by the side of the body. Make a fist and bring the palms to the level of the chest.

Now inhale and extend the right arm in front of you, at the same time bending your left knee and try touching the hip with the toes.

Exhale and repeat with the other arm and leg.

This needs to be done in a continuous motion while inhaling and exhaling through the nostril.

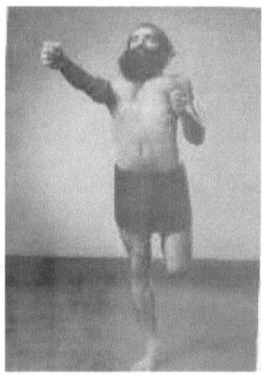

4.4 Yogic Surya Namaskara

Refer to 1.9 for Surya Namaskar with Mantra

4.5 Yogasana

Tadasana

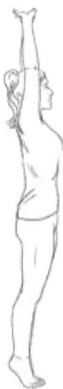

Technique- Stand tall with keeping the feet together and arms by the side of the body.

Inhale and raise your arms above your head. Interlock the fingers and stretch the arms towards the ceiling. Remember to keep the arms behind the ears.

Raise the toes up and gaze at the level of your eyes to maintain balance. Continue breathing and release with an exhale.

Benefits- Improves body balance and posture, Stretches the spine, may help in increasing height if included during the adolescence years, Stimulates the entire nervous system, Adds flexibility to thighs, joints, knees, and ankles.

Contraindication- Low blood pressure, during a headache, as it might worsen, vertigo etc

Hastottanasana

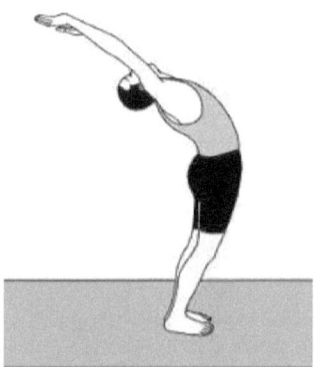

Technique- Stand tall with keeping the feet together and arms by the side of the body.

Inhale and raise your arms above your head and arch your back as much as you can.

Continue breathing and release with an exhale.

Benefits- Improves body balance and posture, Stretches the spine and shoulder, Stimulates the entire nervous system, and opens up the chest hence good for the respiratory system.

Contraindication- Low blood pressure, headache, vertigo, slipped disc, shoulder injury etc.

Vrikshasana

Technique- Stand tall with keeping the feet together and arms by the side of the body.

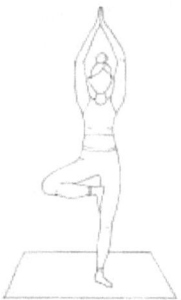

Lift your right foot and place it either below the left knee or above the left knee. Ensure that the right knee is pushed back and in line with hips.

Join the palms to the chest. Once you get the balance right, inhale and raise the arms above your head, while keeping the upper arms behind your ears to maintain a straight upper back. Gaze at the level of the eyes to maintain better balance.

Continue breathing. Release slowly and repeat with the other side.

Benefits- Tones and strengthens the muscles of the leg, Improves balance, mind and body coordination and concentration,

Contraindications- Vertigo, High or low blood pressure, Knee or ankle pain, arthritis, Migraine.

Ardha Chakrasana

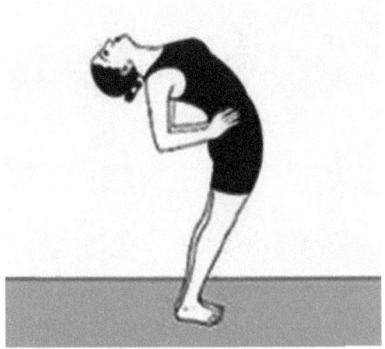

Technique-

- Stand tall with keeping the feet together and arms by the side of the body.
- Inhale and raise your arms above your head while arching the back as much as possible.
- Ensure that your upper arms are behind your ears, this is to ensure proper alignment of the upper back.
- Continue breathing. Release with an exhale.

Benefits- Makes the spine and neck flexible and strengthens the spinal nerves, Improves breathing capacity, Helps in cervical Spondylitis.

Contraindication- Vertigo, Migraine.

Padahastasana

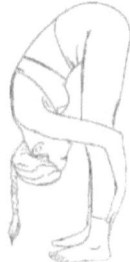

Technique- Stand tall with keeping the feet together and arms by the side of the body.

Inhale and raise the arms above your head, exhaling, and bend forward elongating the back.

The alignment should be- stomach over the thighs, chest over the knees and chin over the shin. Try reaching as low as you can with the palms. The ideal position would be by the side of the feet. Continue breathing and release with an inhale while keeping a straight back.

Benefits- Relaxes neck and shoulders by relieving tension, improves digestion, stretches and strengthens hamstrings and spinal column back muscles, helpful for asthmatic practitioners.

Contraindication- Abdominal inflammation, Hernia, Lower back pain, Pregnancy

Trikonasana

Technique-Stand tall with right foot forward and left foot back. Ensure that the right foot faces forward (parallel to the longer side of the mat) and left foot is parallel to the shorter side of the mat. Also, the right heel should be aligned with the middle of the arch of the left foot.

Now, Inhale and raise the arms sideways, at the level of the shoulders.

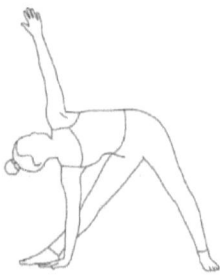

With the next exhalation, bend your body towards the right leg. Try to go as low as possible with the right palm. The ideal position of the palm would be beside the right foot.

Remember this bend should be done while keeping the back straight. Initially, this can be done by standing adjacent to a wall and then bending towards the right. While doing it, the upper back doesn't leave the wall

Look up towards the raised arm. Continue breathing and release with an exhale. Repeat with the other side.

Benefits- Strengthens calf, thigh, and spine, Ideal for Diabetes and constipation management.

Contraindication- Slipped disc, Sciatica, Abdominal surgery, Shoulder injury, Vertigo etc.

Parshva Konasana

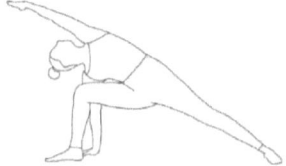

Technique- Stand in the base position of Trikonasana as mentioned above.

Inhale and exhale, bend the right knee, and bend the upper body towards the floor, keeping the right palm beside the right foot.

Stretch the left arm above your head and gaze at the fingers. Keep the pelvis down.

Keep breathing, slowly come out of the posture and repeat the other side. **Benefits-** Excellent posture for legs, pelvis and shoulder strengthing, improves the agility of the body.

Contraindication- Pelvis injury, dizziness, knee pain, shoulder injury, recent abdomen surgery.

Katichakrasana

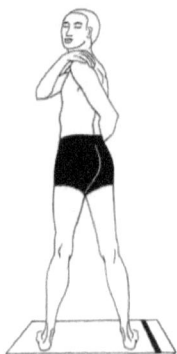

Technique- Stand tall with feet shoulder-width apart, and arms by the side of the body.

Inhale and raise the arms in front of you, up to the level of the shoulders.

With the next exhalation twist your upper body towards the right. To facilitate the twist, place the left palm on the right shoulder.

Continue breathing. Release with an inhale and exhaling repeat the other side.

Benefits- Helps to remove lethargy, improves the flexibility of the spine, opens up the neck and shoulders, helps to relieve back pain.

Contraindication- Hernia, Slip disc, Abdominal inflammation

Dandasana

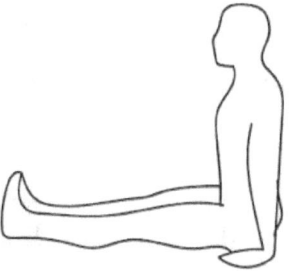

Technique- Sit tall with both legs straightened on the mat and place the palms beside the hips.

Keeping the knees together and feet flexed, press through the palms and keep the elbows straight and straighten the back like a stick.

Benefits- Helps to improve posture and alignment of the body, Lengthens and stretches the spine, shoulders, and chest.

Contraindication- Wrist pain, hip injury, sacrum injury, slipped disc.

Padmasana

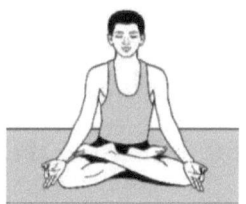

Technique- Sit in crossed leg posture (Sukhasana). Lift your right foot and place it on the left thigh and same with the other foot.

Try to keep the knees on the floor. Keep the back straight and let the palms rest in chin/jnana/bhairava (for males)/bhairavi (for females) mudra.

Benefits- Improves posture, stimulates bladder, spine and pelvis, Stretches the knees, ankles, and hips. Improves concentration and keeps the mind calm and peaceful for meditative practices.

Contraindication- Knee injury, Weak ankle, Spinal injury.

Vajrasana

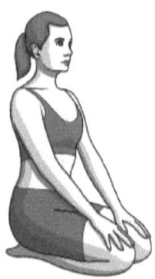

Technique- Start by standing on your knees. Then lower your body in a way that the hips rest on the heels and thighs rest on the calves.

Keep the toes together and heels apart.

Keep the back straight, palms on the knees, and continue breathing. Release slowly.

Benefits- Strengthens pelvic and thigh muscles, Cures digestive acidity and gas formation, and Helps in the treatment of urinary problems.

Contraindication- Knee injury, Arthritis, Weak ankle, Spinal injury.

Yog Mudrasana

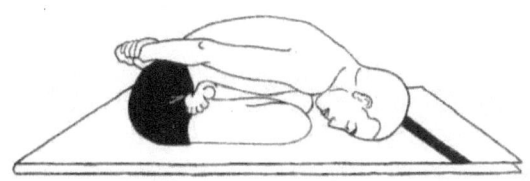

Technique-Sit in Padmasana.

Grab the right wrist with the left palm behind your back. Inhale and exhaling bend forward.

Continue breathing and release with an inhale. Repeat with the other arm.

Yoga Mudra- This is also practiced as Mudra. While practicing this as mudra keep the awareness on the mooladhar Chakra. Inhale and exhaling bend forward, holding the breath in Bahya Kumbhaka.

Inhale and slowly sit up, hold your breath in for a few seconds and focus on the Ajna chakra.

Exhale slowly and move the awareness to the Mooladhar chakra. This is one round, Perform 5-10 rounds.

Benefits- Strengthens back, shoulder, pelvic, and thigh muscles, stimulates abdominal and reproductive organs. On a subtle level, it is used to awaken **Manipura Chakra.** Yoga Mudra is considered excellent preparatory practice for meditation.

Contraindication- Knee injury, Arthritis, Weak ankle, Lower back pain, Pregnancy.

Parvatasana

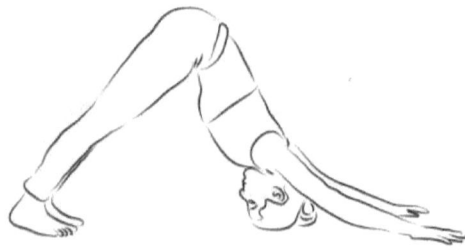

Technique- Come in an all-4 position with shoulder and wrist being in one line, and hips and knees should be in one line too.

Inhale and exhale lift the hips up. Pushing through the shoulders look towards the navel. Keep breathing.

Release by placing the knees on the floor.

Benefits- Stretches the back, shoulder, hamstrings, and calf muscles, improves blood circulation towards the head, relieves the pain in the lower back.

Contraindication- Shoulder injury, wrist injury, recent eye surgery, HBP

Bhadrasana

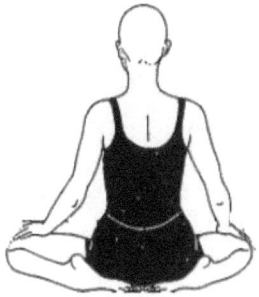

Technique-Sit in Vajrasana and widen the knees as much as possible, while keeping the toes together. Hips should be resting on the floor.

Place the palms on the knees. Breathe normally, Release slowly.

Benefits- Stimulates abdominal organs, ovaries and prostate gland, bladder, and kidneys, Stretches the inner thighs, groins, knees, and heels, soothes menstrual discomfort and sciatica, Consistent practice of this pose until late into pregnancy is said to help ease childbirth.

Contraindication- Groin or knee injury, Ankle injury.

Mandukasana

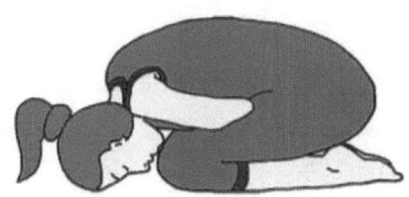

Technique- Sit in Vajrasana, keeping the toes together and heels apart. Now keep your palms in Brahma Mudra and place the palms below the navel.

Inhale and exhaling bend forward, and try to touch the forehead on the ground.

This posture should be done in external retention (Bahya Kumbhak). Release slowly.

Benefits- Relief from diabetes, digestive disorders, and constipation, Improves the flexibility and mobility of the knee and ankle joints.

Contraindication- Peptic or duodenal ulcer, Lower back pain, Knee pain, Abdominal surgery, Ankle injuries.

Ushtrasana

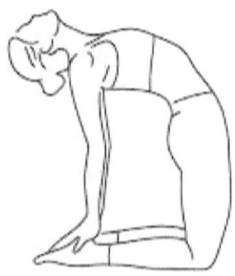

Technique- Stand on your knees.

Inhale and rotate your right arm, and place the right palm over the right heel or wherever you can reach (waist, hamstrings, calves, etc.) Same with the other arm.

Push your hips forward, drop your neck, and continue breathing. Release slowly.

Benefits- Improves digestion, Stretches the chest, back, and shoulders improves posture, and eases menstrual discomfort.

Contraindication- Back injury, Neck injury, High or low blood pressure, vertigo

Shashankasana

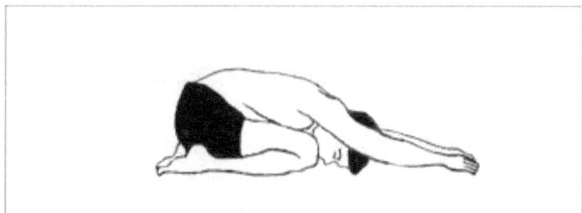

Technique- Sit in Vajrasana with keeping the toes together, heels apart, and back straight.

Inhale, raise your arms above your head and ensure that the spine is upright.

Then exhale and bend forward. Keep the arms on the floor, try touching your forehead on the floor. Continue breathing.

Benefits- Good stretch to the upper body, spine, and shoulders, Massage and stimulates the abdominal muscles and reproductive organs, relieves sciatic pain and menstrual discomfort, compression on the legs can reduce varicose veins.

Contraindication- Knee pain, Neck, Spine, or shoulder injury, Pregnant Women

Uttana Mandukasana

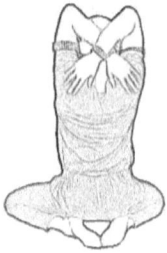

Technique- Sit in Vajrasana and then increase the distance between the knees, while keeping the toes together. Inhale and raise both arms straight up and then cross the palms at the back.

Sit straight, and continue breathing. Release slowly.

Benefits- Strengthens the abdominals, back, shoulders and quadriceps. Opens and increases flexibility in the hips, thighs, knees, shoulders, and chest. Very effective in posture correction, Spontaneously engages the 3 bandhas. Improves the functioning of digestive and excretory systems.

Contraindication- Arthritis, Hernia, Pain in the elbow or shoulder.

Paschimottanasana

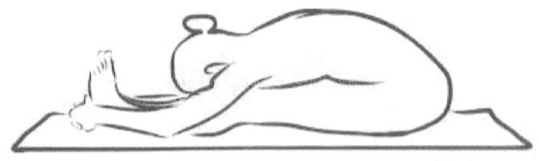

Technique- Sit on your hips with your legs straightened on the mat. Keeping the back straight, inhale and raise your arms above your head.

Exhale and bend forward with an elongated back.

Try reaching with the palms wherever your body allows you to, to calves, to heels, to toes, etc. The alignment should be chest - over the knees, and chin over the shin.

Continue breathing and release with an inhale.

Benefits- Calms the brain and helps relieve stress and fatigue, Stretches the spine, shoulders, and hamstrings. Stimulates the liver, kidneys, ovaries, and uterus. Improves digestion. Relieves menopause and menstrual discomfort.

Contraindication-Lower back pain, Slip Disc, Hernia, Pregnancy.

Purvottanasana

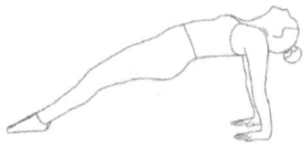

Technique- Sit on your hips with legs straightened on the mat. Slowly, place the palms behind your back with fingers facing backward.

Inhale and exhaling, lift your entire body up while supporting your weight on the palms and on the heels.

Once you are ready try to place the souls of the feet on the floor without bending the knees. Continue breathing and release with an exhale.

Benefits- Strengthens and stretches core, shoulders, chest, triceps, wrists, back, legs, and ankles.

Contraindication- Wrist, neck or shoulder injuries or pain, pregnancy,

Vakrasana

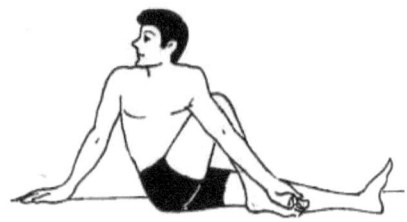

Technique-Sit on your hips with legs straightened on the floor and back straight. Bend your right knee and keep it pulled to the chest.

Inhale and exhaling, place the left palm across the right foot. At the same time, place the right palm behind your back, as close to the body as possible. Keep the elbow straight.

Keeping the back straight, twist your body to the right. continue breathing.

Release slowly and then repeat with the other leg.

Practical

Benefits- Increases the elasticity of the spine and tones the spinal nerves. Massages the abdominal organs, ideal for diabetes management, and Reduces belly fat.

Contraindication- Ulcers, slipped disc, Shoulder or hip injury, pregnancy

Ardha Matsyendrasana

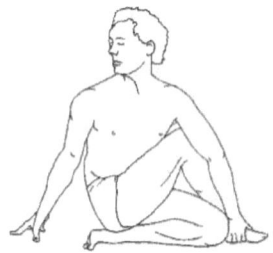

Technique-Begin by sitting on the floor with your legs extended in front of you.

Bend your knees and place your feet flat on the floor, keeping them hip- width apart.

Slide your left foot under your right leg, bringing it to the outside of your right hip. The left knee should be pointing forward.

Cross your right leg over your left leg, placing the right foot on the floor beside the left knee. The right knee should be pointing up toward the ceiling.

Make sure both sitting bones are firmly grounded on the floor.

Inhale and lengthening your spine raise your left arm straight up toward the ceiling.

Exhale and twist your torso to the right, bringing your left elbow to the outside of your right knee. Place your right hand on the floor behind you for support.

Use each inhales to lengthen your spine, and each exhales to deepen the twist, gently turning your gaze over your right shoulder.

Keep your neck relaxed and avoid straining or forcing the twist. Continue breathing.

To release the pose, gently unwind the twist, returning to the starting position.

Repeat the same steps on the opposite side.

Benefits- Improves spinal mobility, stimulates digestion, ideal for diabetes management, improves posture and balance of the body,

Contraindication- Spinal or hip injuries, recent abdominal surgeries, pregnancy, HBP

Gomukhasana

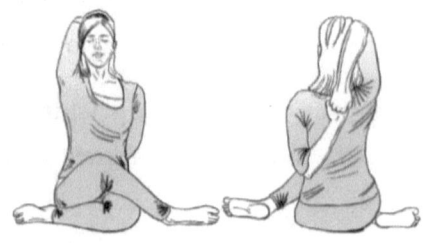

Technique- Sit on the hip and cross your legs in a way that knees are stacked on top of each other and feet come in line with the opposite hips.

Inhale and raise the right arm straight up, bend the elbow, and let the palm reach to the back. At the same time take the left arm from behind the back and try reaching the right palm.

Once you grab the palm, interlock them and continue breathing. Release slowly and repeat with the other arms.

Benefits- Helps to flex the back, making it more elastic. Cures stiff and hunched shoulders. Helps with sciatica and sexual ailments. Helps in diabetes management.

Contraindication- Slipped disc, Weak shoulder, knee, and wrist.

Makarasana

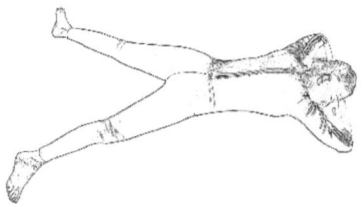

Technique- Lie down on your stomach. Place your palms on top of each other, rest your chin, cheek or forehead on the palms.

Point your toes outwards. Continue breathing.

Alternatively, you can also place your elbows on the floor and let your cheeks rest on the palms.

Benefits- Beneficial in cervical, slipped disc, spondylitis, and sciatica. Very useful in Asthma, knee pain, and other lungs related problems. This pose is best for relaxing after doing an intense sequence.

Contraindication- Pregnancy, Abdominal injury, Hernia, Acid reflux etc.

Bhujangasana

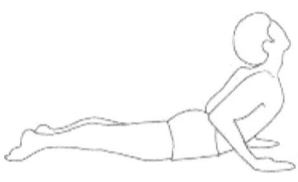

Technique- Lie down on your stomach.

Keep the fingers aligned with the shoulder, elbows touching the body, and forehead on the floor. Inhale and raise the forehead up, chest up, and stomach (only up to the navel) off the floor. While elbows still touch the body.

Continue breathing. Release with an exhale.

Benefits- Strengthens the spine, chest, shoulders, and abdomen, Firms the buttocks, Helps relieve stress and fatigue, Therapeutic for asthma, Traditional texts say that Bhujangasana increases body heat, destroys disease, and awakens kundalini.

Contraindication- Back injury, Carpal tunnel syndrome, Headache.

Shalabhasana

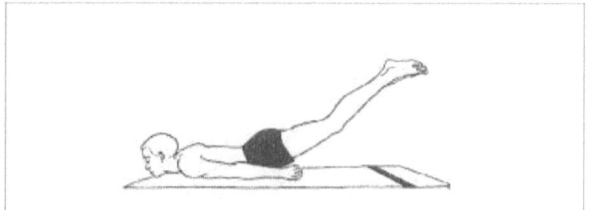

Technique- Lie down on the stomach with your chin on the floor. Keep your palms under the thighs and elbows under the body.

Inhale and exhale, lift your right leg off the floor, without bending the knee. Continue breathing.

Repeat with the other leg. This is called Ekpada - Shalabhasana (One- Legged-Locust-Posture).

Inhale, exhaling lift both the legs off the floor. Release with exhale.

Benefits- It is beneficial in all the disorders at the lower end of the spine as well as sciatica, Removes fat around the abdomen, waist, hips, and thighs. Helpful in managing cervical spondylitis.

Contraindication- Pregnancy, Any recent abdominal surgery, Hernia, Stomach ulcers.

Dhanurasana

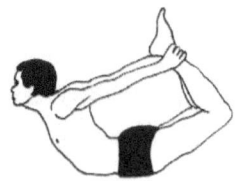

Technique- Lie down on your stomach. Keep the forehead on the floor.

Bend both legs and grab the right heel with the right palm and the left heel with the left palm.

Inhale and bring the forehead, chest, and thighs off the floor. Try to balance yourself on the stomach and then on the pelvis.

Continue breathing. Release with an exhale.

Benefits- Strengthens the back muscles, neck, shoulders, and chest muscles. Stimulates the abdomen and reproductive organs. As per the hatha yoga texts, this is one asana that is very helpful in controlling infertility issues.

Contraindication- Pregnancy, Any recent abdominal surgery, Hernia, Stomach ulcers, Shoulder injury.

Pawanmuktasana

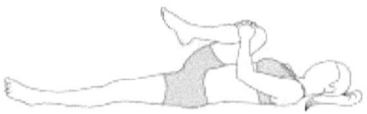

Technique- Lie down on the back.

Inhale and exhale, bring the right knee to the chest, hold it close. Do not strain your neck or shoulders. The other leg stays on the floor.

Repeat with the other leg. This is called Ekpada-Pawan-Muktasana (One- Legged Wind-Release-Posture).

Inhale and exhale, pull both legs towards the chest and hold. If you are ready, you can also lift your neck up (don't strain) and try to touch the nose with the knees.

Continue breathing. Release with an exhale.

Benefits- Relaxes the back and glutes. The pressure on the abdomen releases any trapped gas in the large intestine. The digestive system is improved. Relieves constipation.

Contraindication- Abdominal inflammation, Hernia, Piles, Menstruation, If there is any pain, or stiffness in the neck then head should remain on the floor.

Uttanapadasana

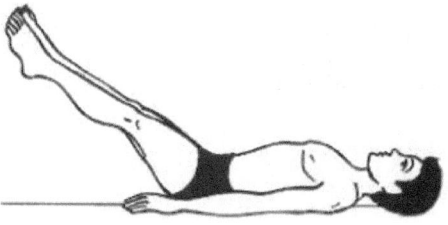

Technique- Lie down on the back. Keep your arms by the side of the hips.

Inhale and exhaling raise both the legs up to an angle of 45 degrees and hold.

Continue breathing and release with an exhale.

Benefits- Tones and strengthens the pelvis, hips, lower back, abdomen, legs, and also the perineum muscles. Reduces fat from the lower abdomen, thighs, and hips. Stimulates the digestive system. Improves the circulation of blood to the lymph nodes in the lower body.

Contraindication- Lower back ache, High BP, Pregnanc

Ardha Halasana

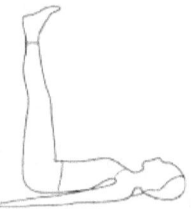

Technique- Lie down on the back. Keep your arms by the side of the hips.

Inhale and exhale, lift your legs up to an angle of 90 degrees. Continue breathing and Release with an exhale.

Benefits- Strengthens the thigh and calf muscles. It reverses the blood flow in the legs, hence has a pain-relieving effect. Alternatively, you can also place the legs against the wall and hold for 5-10 minutes.

Contraindication- Abdominal injury, Hernia, Lower back pain

Setubandhasana

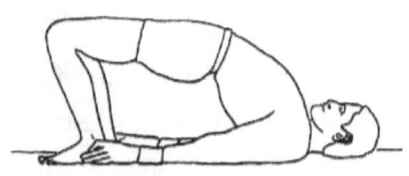

Technique- Lie down on the back. Keep your knees bent and palms by the side of the hips. Inhale, and exhaling lift your hips as high as you can.

If you are ready, try grabbing the heels by the palms. If not, then you can also interlock your fingers, straighten the arms and keep them on the floor.

Continue breathing.

In order to release, find an exhale, release the arms first, and then slowly lower your body.

Benefits- Stretches the chest, neck, and spine. Ideal for relieving lower back pain. Calms the brain and helps alleviate stress. Stimulates

abdominal organs, lungs, and thyroid gland. Improves digestion. Therapeutic for asthma, high blood pressure, osteoporosis, and sinusitis

Contraindication- Neck injury, Cervical.

Saral-Matsyasana

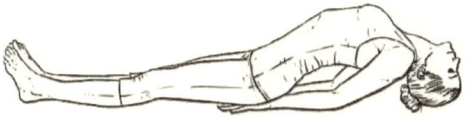

Technique- Lie down on your back. Keep your palms under the hips and elbows under the back.

Now, Inhale and exhale, lift your neck up and look at the toes, hold for 10 seconds and continue breathing. (This step should not be missed, as it prepares your neck for the posture) Slowly bring your neck down.

Now with the next inhalation, lift your neck up once again. And then supporting your weight on the forearms, drop your head on the floor.

The crown should just be touching the floor, your weight shouldn't fall on the crown. Hold for 10 seconds, and continue breathing.

The feet stay together during the whole posture.

Now, find an inhale to lift your neck up, gaze at the toes for a second and slowly drop your back on the floor. Relax.

Benefits- As per Hatha Text Matsyasana is the "destroyer of all diseases." It is the complementary posture after Sarvangasana and Halasana. It Stretches the deep hip flexors (psoas), the muscles (intercostals) between the ribs, the muscles of the belly and throat.

Contraindication- High or low blood pressure, Migraine, Serious lower- back or neck injury.

Shavasana

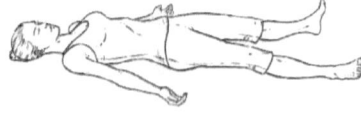

Technique-Lie down on your back. Maintain shoulder width distance between the feet, palms facing the ceiling and eyes closed.

Surrender completely to the gravity, do not resist any pull. Relax with deep conscious breathing.

To release the Shavasana, make movements of the toes, fingers, turn your neck side to side, shift your weight to one side and slowly sit up.

Benefits- Calms the brain and helps relieve stress and fatigue. Helps to lower blood pressure

Contraindication- There are no contraindications as such but in case of Back injury or acute wheezing it would be uncomfortable to lie down like this.

4.6 Preparatory Breathing Practices & Pranayama-

- Sectional Breathing (Abdominal, Thoracic, and Clavicular Breathing)
- Yogic Deep Breathing
- Anuloma Viloma/ Nadi Shodhana
- Concept of Puraka, Rechaka, and Kumbhaka
- Ujjayee Pranayama (Without Kumbhaka)
- Sheetalee Pranayama (Without Kumbhaka)
- Sitkaree Pranayama (Without Kumbhaka)
- Bhramaree Pranayama (Without Kumbhaka)

These will be asked in the demonstration exam. Learn the practice with contraindications and benefits. Refer to Unit 1.12, and Unit 2.7 for the detailed practice.

4.7 Concept and Demonstration of Bandha & Mudra

- Jalandhara Bandha,
- Uddiyana Bandha,
- Mula Bandha,
- Yoga Mudra,
- Maha Mudra,
- Vipreetkarni Mudra

These will be asked in the demonstration exam. Refer to Unit 2.7 for the detailed practice. Prepare with meaning, benefit, and contraindications.

Yoga Mudra can be found in Unit 4.5

4.8 Practices Leading to Dhyan Sadhana

Body awareness and Breath awareness, Yoga Nidra, Antarmauna, Practice of Dhyana

Body and Breath Awareness-

This practice is done at the beginning of the class to build awareness. Consider this practice as a mandate before you begin the class. This simple-looking practice represents the whole idea of going inward.

Different teachers have different styles of doing this practice. It would usually include instructions like these- (Instructions are for standing posture, the same can be done sitting as well)

- Stand tall with both feet together and palms to the chest, and close your eyes.
- Pay attention to your body now. Pay attention to your feet, calves, thighs, pelvis, Spine, Shoulders, palms, neck, and crown.
- Pay attention to the stillness which your body is experiencing right now. Stay with it. (Pause for 10 sec)
- As you build this physical awareness, pay attention to the eye, ensuring the absolute stillness of the eyeballs. The upper eyelid is softly touching the lower eyelid. No Strain. Stay Calm.
- As you build the stillness, pay attention to the breath. Watch the normal flow of inhaling and exhaling. (Pause for 5 sec)
- Watch your breath going in from the nostrils to the throat, to the lungs, to the stomach.
- Feel the coolness of the air as you inhale.
- Watch the breath going out of the stomach, through the lungs, through the throat, and through the nostrils.
- Feel the warmth of the air on your upper lips as you exhale.
- Be aware

Yoga Nidra-

Refer to Chapter 1.15 for the detailed practice.

Antarmauna-

Antarmauna means Inner-Silence.

This is a practice to achieve voluntary control over thoughts and be able to silence them at will. This practice is an integral part of Vipassana meditation in the Buddhist tradition. Antarmauna can be understood as a consequence of regular vipassana meditation.

Antarmauna is also taught by Swami Satyanand Saraswati of the Bihar School Of Yoga. He formulated a 5 steps technique to practice Antar Mauna-

Stage 1: Awareness of external senses

In this stage, the practitioner focuses on sensory perception. It is encouraged to practice this in all aspects of one's day. Such as while sitting, be aware of the touch of the skin against the floor/cloths, be aware of the air you breathe, everything you see, hear, taste, etc. The idea is to be present with the present. This simple-looking practice actually enables the practitioners to shift the focus from gross sensory perceptions to subtle ones.

This practice actually lays down the **foundation of Pratyahara.**

Stage 2: Awareness of the Spontaneous Thought Process

This is the stage of going inward. In this stage, the practitioner focuses on inward thoughts. He / She should now be observing the creation and dissolution of spontaneous thoughts. The idea is to understand the powerlessness of the thought if you don't attach consciousness to it.

Stage 3: Creation and disposal of thoughts at will

In this stage practitioner now creates the thoughts at will and disposes of them at will. This is different from stage 2. Here, spontaneous thoughts are not allowed. The practitioner is training the mind to generate as well as dissolute thoughts with full consciousness.

Stage 4: Awareness and Disposal of Spontaneous Thoughts

Since this is a step-by-step method, one should only try to practice this stage once they have mastered the above stages. In this stage, the practitioner lets the spontaneous thoughts come into the mind with full awareness and disposes of them at will.

When the practitioner masters this stage, a very **strong sense of detachment** from thoughts, builds in them.

Stage 5: Awareness of the Inner Space

This is the stage of being aware of the inner space, without any thoughts. Since now the practitioner can create and stops the thoughts at will, they now stop the thought for a certain period and only observe the inner space or Chidakasha like a blank screen. Eventually, they learn to stop the thoughts for whatever period they want. **This is the final stage of Antarmauna.**

4.9 Concept of Soham/ Hamsa

Recitation of Pranava & Soham

The Yoga ideology attributes the universal sound **Om** to the breathing process. As per yogic science, the easiest way to boost prana shakti with energy is to vibrate it with the **Om sound**. The prana-shakti is metaphorically visualized as **Hamsa (a divine swan that swims in the celestial waters).**

The in-breathing (Poorak) makes the sound **sa** while the out-breathing (Rechaka) makes the sound **ham**. Yogic science says that every individual unconsciously repeats **"ham and sa"** with every respiration. This concept of being unknowingly involved in chanting (generating a sound) is known as **Ajapa - Japa.**

During the practice of dhyana or pranayama, the practitioner is encouraged to focus on these subtle sounds.

As per Yogic science, it usually takes 4 seconds for one round of inhalation-exhalation. And thus, the automatic recital of Hamsa-japa is about 15 times a minute. In one hour- 15*60, it will be 900 repetitions. In one full day-night (or 24 hours) it will be **21,600 repetitions** (900*24).

This mantra is chanted in **two different ways-**

Ham-Sa is chanted by first exhaling and meditating on the word Ham, then inhaling and meditating on the word sa.

So-ham is chanted by first inhaling and meditating on the word So and then exhaling and meditating on the word ham.

When one becomes consciously aware of Hamsa / Soham all the time it is referred to as **Ajapa Gayatri**. It is said that he /she has now mastered Hamsa Vidya and they now hold full control over the prana.

In the non-dualistic sense, the word So-Ham is referred to one's realization of being the self. Sah - He, Aham- I am, Meaning- I am he. He is referred to as the self / Brahma/ higher energy / Purusha Vishesha.

Practice of Dhyana

In the yogic context, **dhyana** is an inward practice, that teaches us to develop control over sensory perception and focus within. Typically, dhyana is done two ways- **With the object and Without the object.**

One chooses the method as per their own choice. In object-oriented practices, one can choose any object they relate to such as any symbol, any deity, sun, candle, etc. The idea is to train the mind to only have thoughts related to the object.

In the object-less dhyana, one usually focuses on the breath, guided commands, chakras, subtle sounds, etc.

The practice of dhyana requires discipline and consistency. Some of the basic rules of practice can be-

- Select a place that is calm, quiet, and free from disturbances.
- Place a soft and thick blanket or pillow, convenient for sitting.
- Sit at ease in any meditative / Sukha asana, and keep the spinal cord straight.
- Close your eyes and mentally see your chosen object.
- Breathe normally and rhythmically in a long inhalation and exhalation
- Consciously keep your focus on the object.

To some, Dhyana strikes as a **boring practice** and they try to avoid it, whereas some only sit with closed eyes, and flow with the mind and later complain that they practice meditation **every day**, yet they have **no control** over themselves. As Yoga practitioners, it is important for us to understand the idea and the **proper technique** behind the practice. It is also **improper** to reject a practice because we **don't want** to put effort into it. It is an undisputed truth that with time, proper technique, and regular practice, the Dhyana becomes **effortless**.

4.10 Methods of Teaching & Evaluation

The basic aim of teaching is to make someone learn. The teacher/instructor arranges the environment for learning and stimulates and guides the student's activities in that environment. The role of the teacher is to teach with utmost effort however, it is the responsibility of students to learn by making honest efforts and grasping the knowledge shared by the teacher.

Teaching methods with special reference to Yoga

Teaching methods can be broadly categorized under 2 categories- **Instructional methods** used in the classroom for teaching **theoretical subjects** and Methods used for teaching **practical skills** in the open air, fields, studios or in gymnasiums, etc.

Traditionally, there have been two approaches to successful teaching: the first is a **teacher-centered approach** and a second is a **student-centered approach.**

The teacher-centered approach is when a teacher demonstrates, shares pros and cons, shares techniques, etc and students only take notes. In the student-centered approach, students participate actively in demonstrations, discussions, etc. In Yoga Learning, **a student-centered approach is highly encouraged.**

Lecture cum demonstration in Yoga: Its meaning, importance, and method of its Presentation

In this method of teaching the teacher performs the practice before the students and simultaneously explains what he/she is doing. He /She also asks relevant questions from the class and students are compelled to observe carefully because they then have to either demonstrate or explain what has been taught.

As compared to other teaching methods such as the Lecture method, Demonstration method, Assignments method, etc, The Lecture cum demonstration method is considered to be the **highly suitable** method for teaching Yoga as it allows participation and attentiveness from both parties.

Seating Plan

The most common seating plan in a yoga class involves – Semi-circular, Circular, Row, and column. These can be utilised wisely as per the size of the group. Such as for the smaller group (7-8 people) Row or semicircular seating may be most effective.

Teaching Aids

Teaching Aids are the props or objects which are used in a Yoga Class, to bring creativity to the class. The most often used aids in a Yoga class are- **Blocks, Belts, Wheels, Sticks, Cushions, etc.**

These aids are mostly used in Asana Practice. Typically props/aids can be used in two ways-

To Supplement the posture- Such as in Paschimottasana, put the bolster/padding below the knee/hips to do a supportive forward bend.

To Enhance the posture- Such as in Paschimottasana, putting the blocks behind the feet and reaching to grab the block instead of the toes.

Role of Language, Voice, Fluency, Clarity, Body, and language (In Teaching)

The information should be conveyed in a language that the students understand. Such as Many students as well as teachers may find Sanskrit to be overwhelming at first, especially foreign students. In such cases, the teacher should try to teach a simple mantra/shloka with a focus on proper pronunciation and meaning. As and when the students become familiar with the sounds, then more mantras and shlokas can be taught.

Along with the language, **voice modulations** are considered to be a great asset in teaching. It is expected that Yoga Teachers have a commanding yet soothing and pleasant voice. Remember that voice doesn't only convey information, it also conveys mood and emotions. Such as-

Whisper - It signals intrigue, mystery, secrets, and more. (Meditation & Relaxation)

Rise and fall - helps maintain interest for all students (Instructions, Explanation)

Louder – Can hear clearly – (Questions, Announcements, and Assignments)

Yelling - shows the teacher has lost control of the situation.

Being fluent in your subject is another important aspect of teaching. Whatever it is you choose to teach, whether it is an Asana, Pranayama, Kriya, or any philosophical topic, anatomical topic, etc., prepare well. Teachers should be able to construct clear thoughts and be able to convey them effectively. Their preparation reflects in their voice.

The body language of Yoga Teachers says a lot about their personality, confidence, and bond with the students. Sitting with a slouching back while taking a class, rolling eyes at incorrect answers, being Unable to make proper eye contact, annoyed facial expressions, too much or robotic hand gestures, etc can take the interest away from the class, **despite the teacher being knowledgeable.**

Preparation for a Yoga Class (Before & After)

Before the pandemic, all the learning happened in person. But ever since the pandemic a world of digitalization opened up and Online classes took over. The prep for an online class vs an in-person class is different in certain ways.

The Prep of Online Class

- Before the class begins, ensure that you have a good internet connection, the device is fully charged or connected to a charger.
- Keep your background/sitting area clean/uncluttered. Ensure that you are visible to the students.
- In Online class scenarios, **the instructions** you give play a very important role. Be very thorough and clear. Most of the time you would just be watching and giving instructions. There would be **no opportunity to do a "Follow me" routine** for the entire duration. So be very clear with giving instructions
- Plan your routine ahead but if you are taking a group class, you may need to be proactive in changing the asanas depending upon the receptivity of the students. Since you are not

physically present there, there is no assistance. So be **patient and proactive.**
- If you must, then introduce props like belts, and yoga blocks in the class. These are very helpful in an online /offline setting.
- Before you introduce any kriyas, gain the confidence of the students. Ensure that they are not overwhelmed.
- Do not introduce advanced kriyas until you are very sure that students are good with the basic ones. For Instance- Before introducing sutra neti, ensure that the student is proficient with Jala neti.

The Prep of Offline Class

- It is appropriate to take the class in an atmosphere where there is no pollution, and the air is fresh and clean.
- For every practitioner 6*3 places are needed to sit and lie on the floor while doing asana or practice. Mats should be placed in the classroom or the practitioner should bring them along with him.
- The physical presence of a teacher in the classroom definitely gives confidence to the students as you would be able to provide assistance with the student's consent.

After the class

- Always end the class with a prayer/ OM chanting/ Affirmations
- Once the class is over, ask students if they have any questions.
- Ask for their experiences.
- **Learning is a two-way approach.** Ensure the practitioner's need is addressed, Ensure that they are equally involved.

Question / Answer sessions and Feedback sessions will ensure that the practice is going in the right direction.

Lesson plan

A lesson plan is a teacher's daily guide for what students need to learn, how it will be taught, and how learning will be measured. A good lesson plan should be prepared shortly before the use. It should be specific and detailed. Keeping the lesson plan ready is essential for Yoga Teachers as it shows commitment of the teacher.

It also helps the teacher to decide the correct technique/sequence for the class. Teachers will also be able to time the class better.

A lesson plan should include:

- Statement of objectives of the session.
- Statement of materials needed such as blocks, belts, partners, etc.
- Description of method and procedures to be used such as while asking the practitioners to hold the asana whether the focus would be on giving the numeric counts or counting the breath etc
- Provisions for connecting previous and future practices. This approach is really helpful in building strength and improving flexibility. In disease management, building on to the previous practice remains the fundamental practice.
- Provisions for questions/discussions after the lesson. This practice helps in strengthening the teacher-practitioner bond. Practitioners can give feedbacks/suggestions which can be utilized in further classes.

Sequence of Teaching

- Setting the atmosphere suitable for the session by prayer / Body and breath awareness.
- Introduction to the practice
- Verbal Instruction
- Demonstrations
- Analysing the whole performance as a whole as well as in stages.
- Detection & Correction of mistakes in the performance.
- Giving Instructions with emphasis on salient points.
- Repeat demonstrations with clear explanations of the various stages involved.
- Complete rest in Shavasana at the end.
- Sum up points covered and Question/Answer session.
- Self-Evaluation by the teacher

Presentation of lessons in specific Yogic practices: Kriya, Asana, Pranayama, and Dhyana.

Suitable lesson plan for Pranayama / Kriya-

Introduction of the practice, Demonstration, Limitations, and Benefits, Individual/Group practice, Relaxation

Suitable lesson plan for Dhyana –

Introduction of the practice, Instructions, Relaxation

Suitable lesson plan for Asana-

Prayer, Sukshma Vyayama, Surya Namaskara, Asana Sequence as per the strength level of the individual/group, Shavasana.

In general physical practices should follow the structure of - Instruction, Silent demonstration, Observation, Correction, and encouragement

Assessment of a Yoga class (detection and correction of mistakes)

The term assessment refers to the wide variety of methods that educators use to evaluate, measure, and document the academic readiness, learning progress, and skill acquisition of students. In a Yoga class, assessments can be implemented to evaluate students' preparation and learning at any stage.

- Assessing a student's progress will help teachers understand what the students know, understand, and are able to do.
- Assessment is very important in order to track progress, plan the next steps, and evaluate overall learning objectives. A yoga class may be assessed based on below mentioned parameters-

Posture alignment, Breathing pattern, Follow-up practices, Maintenance, Gradual progression toward perfection and Awareness etc.

MULTIPLE CHOICE QUESTIONS

Q1. What is the origin of the word "Yoga"?

a. Yuj, b. Yujir, c. Yog, d. Yogasya

Q2. Yuj Samyoga means-

a. To unite, b. To integrate, c. To restrain, d. To discriminate

Q3. "Yoga-chitta-vritti-nirodhah" This definition of Yoga is given by-

a. Bhagwad Gita, b. Patanjali, c. Ved Vyasa, d. Lord Shiva

Q4. "yoga uchyate"?

a. Karmah, b. Samatvam, c. Kaushlam, d. Chitta

Q5. "Buddhi-yukto jahātīha ubhe sukṛita-duṣhkṛite, tasmād yogāya yujyasva yogaḥ karmasu kauśhalam " This shloka is from which chapter of Bhagavad Gita?

a. 2.50, b. 2.48, c. 2.45, d. 2.40

Multiple Choice Questions

Q6. yuktāhāra-vihārasya yukta-cheṣhṭasya (BG 6.17). What is the meaning of the word "yukta"?

a. Moderate, b. Limitless, c. Less, d. Very less

Q7. As per the texts, the ultimate objective of Yoga is –

a. Samadhi, b. Health, c. Spirituality, d. Moral values

Q8. Yoga is physical exercise- True or False.

a. False, b. True

Q9. Panini was a –

a. Grammarian, b. Yoga Guru, c. Shiva's disciple, d. Patanjali's Guru

Q10. The union of the Jeevatma (individual self) with the Paramatma (the universal self) is referred as-

a. Samadhi, b. Yog, c. Bliss, d. Santosha

Q11. The earliest known record of Yoga is Bhagavad Gita-

a. False, b. True

Q12. Ayurveda is part of -

a. Rig Veda, b. Sama Veda, c. Yajur Veda, d. Atharva Veda

Q13. Jnana Kanda is also known as-

a. Up-Veda, b. Upanishad, c. Vedanga, d. None of the above

Multiple Choice Questions

Q14. The knowledge of Yoga didn't exist before the Vedic period.

a. True, b. False

Q15. Which statement is correct?

a. Upanishads are stand-alone scripture, b. Upanishads are part of Vedas, c. a&b, Both, d. None of the above

Q16. The commentary of PYS by Veda Vyasa is known as-

a. Yoga Sutra, b. Yoga Bhashya, c. Yoga Rahasya, d. Sutra

Q17. Patanjali Yoga Sutra is the contemporary text of-

a. Bhagavad Gita, b. Upanishad, c. Hatha Yoga Pradipika, None of the above

Q18. Who is known as the father of modern yoga?

a. Patanjali, b. Lord Krishna, c. Adi Yogi, d. Nath Yogi

Q19. "Viniyog Hatha Yoga" lineage is started by

a. Shri Krishnamacharya, b. Jiddu Krishnamurti, c. BKS Iyengar, d. Pattabhi Jois

Q20. Parliament of Religion was held in -

a. 1894, b. 1893, c. 1890, d. 1895

Q21. Taking a bath immediately after yoga is highly recommended.

a. True, b. False

Q22. One of the prime reasons Yogic practices are different than other exercise formats is-

a. Movement and breath coordination, b. Ensuring the clean environment, c. inclusion of prayer / mantra, d. Usage of the mat

Q23. Bhujangasana is a relaxing posture and a yoga class can end with Bhujangasana.

a. False, b. True

Q24. The correct way of releasing the posture is -

a. Last in first out, b. First in last out, c. Depending upon the convenience, d. A and C

Q25. In modern times, Kriya Yoga is primarily taught by-

a. Paramahansa Yogananda, b. Swami Vivekananda, c. Maharishi Mahesh Yogi, d. Swami Sivananda Saraswati

Q26. Who was the guru of Gorakshanath?

a. Matsyendranath, b. Lord Shiva, c. Maharishi Patanjali, d. Sage Marichi

Q27. "Interest is the best motivation for learning" - is this statement correct?

a. Yes, b. No

Q28. A. In order to master Asana, it is very important to keep pushing your limits without worrying about injuries.

b. Practicing Asanas consistently with relaxed efforts will eventually lead to perfection.

Which statement is true?

a. A & B both, b. B, c. A, d. None of the above

Q29. Dhyana is -

a. Concentration. b. Meditation, c. Dharana, d. None of the above

Q30. A minimum gap between eating and practice should be-

a. 15-30 minutes, b. 1 hour. c. 2 hours, d. 40 minutes

Q31. When did Swami Vivekanada go to the parliament of religion?

a. 11th Sep 1893, b. 11th Nov 1893, c. 11th Dec 1893, d. 12th Jan 1893

Q32. The style of Yoga taught by Swami Aurobindo is known as-

a. Integral yoga, b. Kriya Yoga, c. Mauna Yoga, d. Hot Yoga

Multiple Choice Questions

Q33. Who was the guru of Swami Dayanand Saraswati?

a. Swami Virajanand Dandasheesha, b. Swami Kuvalyananda, c. Swami Ramkrishna Paramhansa, d. Swami Aurobindo

Q34. Swami Vivekananda was born on -

a. 12th Jan 1863, b. 12th Sep 1863, c. 12th Jan 1864, d. 12th Jan 1865

Q35. Brahma Samaja was established by -

a. Raja Rammohan Roy, b. Swami Vivekananda, c. Swami Dayananda Saraswati, d. Swami Aurobindo

Q36. Satyartha Prakasha is written by -

a. Swami Dayananda Saraswati, b. Swami Ramakrishna Paramhansa, c. Swami Dipankara, d. Swami Aurobindo

Q37. Arya Samaj is established by-

a. Swami Dayananda Saraswati, b. Swami Ramakrishna Paramhansa, c. Swami Dipankara, d. Swami Aurobindo

Q38. Awake, Arise, and ....

a. Keep walking, b. Stop not until the goal has been achieved, c. Never turn back, d. None of the above

Q39. One of the main teachings by Maharshi Raman is -

a. Silence, b. Kriya Yoga, c. Bhakti, None of the above

Multiple Choice Questions

Q40. The mother of Vivekananda is-

a. Bhuvaneshwari Devi, b. Sundaramma, c. Yashoda Bai, d. Swarnalata Devi

Q41. The three stages of Jnana Yoga are-

a. Shravana, Pramana, Nididhyasana, b. Shravana, Manana, Nididhyasana, c. Manana, Shravana, Nididhyasana, d. Shravan, Smriti, Nididhyasana

Q42. Which of the following helps in Jnana Yoga -

a. Antahkarana Chatushtaya, b. Sadhana Chatushtaya, c. Purushartha Chatushtaya, d. None of the above

Q43. The meaning of Uparati is -

a. Withdrawal of senses, b. Control of senses, c. Endurance, d. Control of mind

Q44. The ultimate objective of practicing Jnana Yoga is -

a. Moksha, b. Discrimination between real and unreal, c. Knowledge of Self, d. All of the above

Q45. Match the following-

Sama —--- Withdrawal of senses

Dama   Control of senses

Titiksha   Calming the mind

Uparati   Patience

a. a-c b-b c-d d-a, b. a-c b-a c-d d-b, c. a-a b-b c-c d-d, d. a-a b-c c-b d-a

Q46. Subheccha is the first step to developing detachment in a Jnana Yogi.

a. True, b. False

Q47. Which one is not part of Sapta Bhumika?

a. Subheccha, b. Padārtha Bhavana, c. Turia, d. Mumukshutva

Q48. In Sapta Bhumika, which stage makes the mind thin like a thread?

a. Tanumanasi, b. Vicharana, c. Sattva Patti, d. None of the above

Q49. Which one is not part of Shad Sampat.

a. Sama, b. Titiksha, c. Kama, d. Uparati

Q50. Moksha is attained in -

a. Turiya, b. Padārtha Bhavana, c. Sattva Patti, d. Tanumanasi

Q51. "health as a state of complete physical, mental and social well-being and not merely the absence of disease or infirmity" - This definition of health is given by -

a. WHO, b. AIIMS, c. International Medical Association, d. Cancer Research Institute

Q52. Yoga is an excellent discipline to produce mental health but can not be called a preventive measure against physical ailments.

a. True, b. False

Multiple Choice Questions

Q53. Yogic practices should not be attempted during pregnancy.

a. True, b. False, c. Some practices need to be definitely avoided such as agnisar kriya., d. A & C

Q54. Yogic practices along with adequate diet habits can be the best way to maintain health.

a. True, b. False, c. May be, d. Not Really

Q55. Dassyam is one of the "Types of Bhaktas" as per Bhagavad Gita-

a. True, b. False.

Q56. Dhyana practices help to strengthen -

a. Vijnanamaya Kosha, b. Annamaya Kosha, c. Pranamaya Kosha, d. None of the above

Q57. Which of these can be klishta Vritti

a. Pratyaksha, b. Pramana, c. Agama, d. All of the above

Q58. Kleshas can be kept in a weak state by practicing -

a. Ashtanga Yoga, b. Pratipaksha Bhavna, c. Kriya Yoga, d. Yama and Niyama

Q59. Stubborn attachment to sense objects is referred as-

a. Avirati, b. Bhranti-Darshan, c. Alabdha - Bhumikatva, d. Anavasthitattva

Multiple Choice Questions

Q60. The practice of _____ Kumbhak is suggested to have a calming effect on the mind in PYS.

a. Bahya Kumbhaka, b. Antar Kumbhaka, c. Kevala Kumbhaka, d. Bandha with Kumbhaka

Q61. Which mudra is performed in Basti Kriya

a. Pashini Mudra, b. Khechari Mudra, c. Ashwini Mudra, d. Moola Bandha

Q62. Laukiki is -

a. Another name of Nauli, b. Another name of Basti, c. Kriya mentioned in Hatha Ratnavali, d. Trataka

Q63. One of the major contraindication for Kapalbhati is -

a. Gastric Ulcer, b. Detached Retina, c. Epilepsy, d. All of the above

Q64. The length of the cloth in Dhauti Kriya is -

a. One and a half meter, b. One meter, c. At Least 2 meter, d. None of the above

Q65. In Dhauti kriya, the cloth can be left in the stomach for-

a. 3 minutes, b. 3-5 minutes, c. 5-20 minutes, d. Minimum 30 minutes

Q66. Another name for Shankha Prakshalana is -

a. Varisara, b. Vatsara, c. Vanisara, d. Plavini

Q67. The asana used in Shankha Prakshalana Kriya is -

a. Ardha Chakrasana, b. Pada Hastasana, c. Matsyendrasana, d. Udarakarshanasana

Q68. For best results Shatkarma should be done first thing in the morning after Pranayama.

a. True, b. False

Q69. Which Kriya is referred to as "Goddess of creation" ?

a. Nauli, b. Trataka, c. Plavini, d. None of the above

Q70. Twenty kinds of disease caused by excess mucus are destroyed through the effect of which karma ?

a. Dhauti, b. Basti, c. Kapalabhati, d. Nauli

Q71. Sukshma Vyayama was designed and propagated by

a. Maharishi Kartikeya Maharaj of Himalaya, b. Dheerendra Brahmchari, c. Sage Swatmarama, d. Sage Gheranda

Q72. Sukshma Vyayama is only applicable for senior practitioners

a. True, b. False

Q73. Sthula Vyayama can be understood as-

a. Isolated movements, b. Compound movements, c. Cardio movements, d. B &C

Multiple Choice Questions

Q74. In traditional Surya Namaskara which Asana is done only once per leg-

a. Ashtanga Namaskara, b. Bhujangasana, c. Parvatasana, d. A & B both

Q75. Surya Namaskara originates from Hatha Yoga Pradipika

a. True, b. False

Q76. The mantra for "Prostration to him who produces everything".

a. Om Savitre Namah, b. Om Pushne Namah, c. Om Hiranyagarbhaya Namah, d. Om Suryaya Namah

Q77. Would you recommend Surya Namaskar to a practitioner with back pain?

a. Not at all, b. A variation can be suggested, c. Yes, Surya Namaksar has no relation with the back pain, d. None of the above

Q78. Om Ravaye Namah means-

a. Prostration to him who is the cause of all changes, b. Prostration to him who diffuses light, c. Prostration to him who is fit to be worshiped, d. Prostration to him who is the cause of all luster.

Q79. What is the most suggested set of movements for injury rehabilitation?

a. Sukshma Vyayama, b. Sthula Vyayama, c. Surya Namaskara, d. A & B

Multiple Choice Questions

Q80. Sukshma Vyayama consist of -

a. 50 movements, b. 48 movements, c. 47 movements, d. 52 movements

Q81. As per Hatha Text Asana practice brings

a. Sthirta (Stability), b. Dhridhta (Strength), c. Sithilta (Flexibility), d. Laghatvam (Lightness)

Q82. As per Patanjali, dualities can be overcome by practicing-

a. Pranayama, b. Karma Yoga, c. Asana, d. Chitta Prasadanam

Q83. In total there are-

a. 32 Asana, b. 84 Lakhs Asana, c. 15 Asana, d. 84 Asana

Q84. In Yoga Sutra, Asanas have been given importance because-

a. It would prepare the practitioner to sit in meditation for a longer duration, b. It would help the practitioner to overcome dualities, c. It is the prime eligibility for pratyahara, d. A & B

Q85. In Hatha Yoga, Asana are treated important because-

a. Only when the body is healthy, Raja yoga can be achieved, b. Only when the body is healthy, control of the mind can be achieved, c. Its not given importance, Dhyan is given much more importance than asana, d. A & B

Multiple Choice Questions

Q86. Mastering the asana is only possible in kumbhakas.

a. True, b. False, one should not hold the breath unless otherwise instructed.

Q87. Asana is a very recent aspect of Yoga practice.

a. True,, b. False, Asanas are one of the core aspects of Yoga Practice.

Q88. Just like Surya Namskara, Every asana should be accompanied by respective mantras

a. True, b. False

Q89. What are the 5 parameters of fitness?

a. Cardiovascular fitness, Strength, Stamina, Flexibility, Body balance

b. Cardiovascular fitness, Lungs Health, Blood Quality, Bone Health, Hormonal Health

c. Agility, Strength, Fat content, Muscle content, Stamina

d. None of the above

Q90. HYP mentions-

a. 15 asana, b. 32 asana, c. 84 Asana, d. As many asana as there are species.

Q91. Bhakti Yoga is not for householders. It is a path for Sanyasins.

a. True, b. False

Q92. Which is not a part of navvidha Bhakti

a. Archanam, b. Kirtanam, c. Danam, d. Pada-Sevanam

Q93. Nav Vidha Bhakti is mentioned in

a. Narada Bhakti Sutra, b. Bhagawag Gita, c. Ramayana, d. Bhagawat Purana

Q94. The desirer of the wealth is referred as which type of bhakta?

a. Artharthee, b. Arta, c. Greedy, d. Jigyasu

Q95. Which type of devotee is considered best by Shri Krishna?

a. Jnani, b. Jigyasu, c. Artharthee, d. Arta

Q96. Mirabai was part of the -

a. Bhakti Yoga Path, b. Karma Yoga Path, c. Jnana Yoga Path, d. Hatha Yoga Path

Q97. Pooraka is

a. Inhalation, b. Exhalation, c. Retention, d. None of the above

Q98. Yoga is

a. Union of individual self and supreme self, b. Exercise, c. Spiritual movement, d. None of the above

Multiple Choice Questions

Q99. Patanjali defines yoga as-

a. Yogaschittavrittinirodhah, b. Samatvam Yogah Uchyate, c. Yogah Karma Kaushalam, d. Union of individual self and supreme self

Q100. Which is path is suggested as the surest way to achieve liberation in Kali Yuga

a. Bhakti Yoga, b. Karma Yoga, c. Jnana Yoga, d. Raja Yoga

Q101. What is the Beeja Mantra for vayu?

a. Yam, b. Ram, c. Tham, d. Lam

Q102. According to the Bhagavad Gita, people should aspire to do which type of Karma?

a. Shukla - Karma, b. Krishna - Karma, c. Shukla - Krishna, d. Ashukla - Akrishna

Q103. Karma yoga is the path for students only -

a. True, b. False

Q104. Which is the prime scripture of Karma Yoga

a. Bhagwad Gita, b. Bhagawat Purana, c. HYP, d. GS

Q105. The prime concept of Karma Yoga is to -

a. Stay detached from the consequences of your actions., b. Take responsibility for your actions, c. Always do good karma, d. All of the above

Multiple Choice Questions

Q106. Yogah……..kaushalam.

a. Karmasu, b. Samatvam, c. Chitta, d. Uparati

Q107. The concept of Karma teaches that you are the reason for your action.

a. True, b. False

Q108. One has full right to actions but is not entitled to the fruits of actions.

a. True, b. False

Q109. Krishan says that path of inaction is superior.

a. True, b. False

Q110. Which is correct in the context of Karma Yoga

a. Human beings are bound to act due to their inherent nature, b. Inaction is a superior way, c. One should take responsibility for their actions and the consequences, d. You are sometimes entitled to the fruits of your action

Q111. Karma Yoga may be hard to implement in today's time but once implemented it is the easiest way to let go of the ego and attain mental peace.

a. True, b. False

Q112. The word "Ayama" in Pranayama means-

a. To stretch, b. To hold, c. To breath, d. To let go

Multiple Choice Questions

Q113. Prana can be understood as oxygen

a. True, b. False

Q114, "Ascension" is a process of

a. Udana, b. Apana, c. Samana, d. Vyana

Q115. The Prana responsible for Yawning is -

a. Naga, b. Devdutta, c. Dhananjaya, d. Kurma

Q116. Dhyana is actually a transcendental stage which happens as a result of continuous practice of Pratyahara and Dharna.

a. True, b. False

Q117. The hunger inhibiting hormone is -

a. Leptin, b. Insulin, c. Glucagon, d. None of the above

Q118. As per Swatmarama, regular practice of Nadi shodhana can purify the nadis within-

a. 3 months, b. 3 years, c. 2 months, d. 2-3 months

Q119. Which is the most suggested Asana for Pranayama as per HYP?

a. Padmasana, b. Siddhasana, c. Vajrasana', d. Ardha Padmasana

Q120. Kapalbhati is -

a. A pranayama, b. A kriya

Q121. The elements of Pranayama are-

a. Puraka, Rechaka, Kevala, b. Puraka, Rechaka, Kumbhaka, c. Puraka, Bahya Kumbhaka, Antar Kumbhaka, d. None of the above

Q122. Which one is the throat lock ?

a. Jalandhara bandha, b. Uddiyana Bandha, c. Moola Bandha, d. Maha Bandha

Q123. Uddiyana Bandha is done in which breathing?

a. Bahya Kumbhaka, b. Antar Kumbhaka, c. Rechaka, d. Pooraka

Q124. Jalandhara Bandha is done in which breathing?

a. Bahya Kumbhaka, b. Antar Kumbhaka, c. Rechaka, d. A & B both

Q125. Moola Bandha is done in which breathing?

a. Bahya Kumbhaka, b. Antar Kumbhaka, c. Rechaka, d. A & B both

Q126. Maha Bandha is done in which breathing?

a. Bahya Kumbhaka, b. Antar Kumbhaka, c. Rechaka, d. A & B both

Q127. Pregnant women can do which practice?

a. Jalndhara Bandha, b. Uddiyana Bandha, c. Maha Bandha, d. None of the above

Q128. Agni Sara kriya is the preparatory practice for which bandha?

a. Jalndhara Bandha, b. Uddiyana Bandha, c. Maha Bandha, d. Moola Bandha

Q129. Cervical Spnodylosis is contraindicatory for which bandha?

a. Jalndhara Bandha, b. Uddiyana Bandha, c. Maha Bandha, d. A & C Both

Q130. Which bandha induces hyperactivity?

a. Jalndhara Bandha, b. Uddiyana Bandha, c. Maha Bandha, d. Moola Bandha

Q131. Which bandha helps in holding the nectar in vishuddhi chakra?

a. Jalndhara Bandha, b. Uddiyana Bandha, c. Moola Bandha, d. None of the above

Q132. Dhyan is a state of Thoughtless-ness

a. True, b. False

Q133. Dhyan is .... Flow of mind towards the chosen object.

a. Random, b. Uninterrupted, c. Interrupted, d. None of the above

Q134. Breath Observation can be a Dhyana Technique.

a. True, b. False

Q135. Dhyana is which limb of Ashtanga Yoga?

a. 3, b. 4, c. 7, d. 8

Q136. Dharna means-

a. Concentration, b. Meditation, c. Withdrawal of unwanted senses, d. Transcendetal State

Q137. Dhyan and Dharana are interchangeable terms. They mean the same thing.

a. True, b. False

Q138. To induce the opposite of thought in case of a negative thought comes in is referred as-

a. Mindfulness Meditation, b. Pratipaksha Bhavana, c. Aparigraha, d. Ishwara Pranidhana

Q139. Dhyana helps in -

a. Improving intuitions, b. Relaxing mind, c. Being observant, d. All of the above

Q140. Dhyana is contraindicatory practice for -

a. Pregnancy, b. HBP, c. Epilepsy, d. Depression

Q141. Vibhuti Pada contains-

a. 34 Sutra, b. 55 Sutra, c. 51 Sutra, d. 31 Sutra

Q142. Samadhi Pada is about -

a. Contemplation, b. Practice, c. Properties & Power, d. Liberation

Multiple Choice Questions

Q143. tadā draṣṭuḥ_____vasthānam ?

a. Svarūpe, b. Rupe, c. Chittah, d. Ishwara

Q144. śabda-jñāna-anupātī _____vikalpaḥ?

a. Vastu-śūnyo, b. Abhava, c. Agamah, d. Vastu

Q145. abhyāsa_____ tannirōdhaḥ

a. Vairāgyābhyām, b. Pranidhana, c. Anushasanam, d. Itaratra

Q146. _____mithyā-jñānam-atadrūpa pratiṣṭham.

a. Viparyayo, b. Vikalpah, c. Pramana, d. Nidra

Q147. abhāva pratyayālambanā vṛitti_____

a. Nidrā, b. Smrtih, c. Pratyaksham, d. None of the above

Q148. anu-bhūta-viṣaya_____ smṛtiḥ

a. Pramosah, b. Asampramoṣaḥ, c. Alambana, d. Avikalpah

Q149. vṛttayaḥ pañcatayyaḥ_____

a. Kliṣṭākliṣṭāḥ, b. Klista, c. Aklista, d. All of the above

Q150. pramāṇa viparyaya _____nidrā smṛtayaḥ

a. Vikalpa, b. Itaratra, c. Nirodhah, d. None of the above

Q151. karmaṇy-evādhikāras te mā _____kadāchana

a. Phaleshu, b. Karmeshu, c. Akarmani, d. Yoga

Q152. yoga-sthaḥ kuru karmāṇi saṅgaṁ tyaktvā dhanañjaya siddhy-asiddhyoḥ samo bhūtvā samatvaṁ yoga uchyate

This shloka is from which chapter of Bhagavad Gita ?

a. 2.48, b. 2.47, c. 2.50, d. 2.49

Q153. Skill in _____ is yoga.

a. Action, b. Balance, c. Success, d. Equanimity

Q154. "Yogah Karmashu Kaushalam " is the excerpt from which chapter of Bhagavad Gita?

a. 2.50, b. 2.48, c. 2.50, d. 6.14

Q155. "Samatvam Yog Uchyate" means-

a. Not be attached to action, b. Equanimity is called Yog, c. This is called Yog, d. None of the above

Q156. The core teaching of Bhagavad Gita remains overcoming the duality of pleasure/pain, success / failure, Profit /Loss etc.

a. True, b. False

Q157. mā te saṅgo 'stv-_____

a. Akarmaṇi, b. Karmani, c. Karmeshu, d. None of the above

Q158. As per Bhagavad Gita, one should discard reward seeking behavior. As this will bind the individual with the results, good or bad.

a. True, b. False

Q159. How many chapters are there in Bhagavad Gita-

a. 16, b. 18, c. 12, d. 20

Q160. Bhagavad Gita is a conversation between -

a. Shri Krishna and Arjuna, b. Sanjaya and Dhritarashtra, c. Shri Krishna and the world, d. Shri Krishna and the Abhimanyu

Q161. Who is the author of Hatha Yoga Pradipika

a. Sage Swatmaram Suri, b. Sage Gheranda, c. Sage Matsyendranath, d. Sage Kuvalayananda

Q162. Which Asana is considered the most important asana in HYP

a. Padmasana, b. Bhadrasana, c. Siddhasana, d. Vajrasana

Q163. Which asana is not mentioned in HYP ?

a. Veerasana, b. Bhujangasana, c. Paschimottanasana, d. Shavasana

Q164. Prayasa is mentioned as one of the -

a. Sadhaka Tattva (Cause of Success), b. Badhaka Tattva (Cause of Failure), c. Practice of Nauli, d. None of the above

Multiple Choice Questions

Q165. Basti is done in which Asana

a. Utkatasana, b. Malasana, c. Mandukasana, d. None of the above

Q166. Which pranayama helps in removing the worms?

a. Kapalbhati, b. Suryabhedi, c. Ujjayi, d. Bhastrika

Q167. Which mudra is performed during Sheetali Pranayama?

a. Khechari Mudra, b. Kaki Mudra, c. Ashwini Mudra, d. A & B both

Q168. In Kapalbhati air is inhaled and exhaled repeatedly through the nostrils like a pair of bellows being pumped.

a. True, b. False

Q169. Match the following -

Arambha - Avastha (Beginning Stage)	kettledrum
Gatha- Avastha (Vessel Stage)	drum
Parichaya - Avastha (Stage of Increase)	flute, veena
Nishpatti - Avastha (Stage of consummation)	tinkling sound

a. A- D, B- A, C-B, D-C, b. A- A, B- D, C-B, D-C, c. A- C, B- A, C-D, D-B, d. A- D, B- A, C-C, D-D

Multiple Choice Questions

Q170. Vipareeta Karani is type of

a. Asana, b. Mudra, c. Bandha, d. Sthula Vyayama

Q171. What is Prasthantrayi?

a. The Upanishads, the Bhagavad Gita and the Brahma Sutras, b. The Upanishads, the Bhagavad Gita and the Vedas, c. The Upanishads, Shad Darshana and the Brahma Sutras, d. None of the above

Q172. Which one is known as Sruti Prasthan?

a. The Brahma Sutra, b. The Upanishad, c. Samkhya, d. Shad Darshana

Q173. Which is known as Yukti Prasthan?

a. Bhagavad Gita, b. Nyaya Darshana, c. Vedanta, d. None of the above

Q174. In the context of Prasthan Trayi, Bhagavad Gita is also referred as-

a. Shruti Prasthana, b. Smriti Prasthana, c. Yukti Prasthana, d. Karma Yoga Shastra

Q175. Which karma should be kept hidden like a golden casket?

a. Trataka, b. Basti, c. Bahishkrit, d. Moola Shodhan

Q176. Epileptics should not do Trataka.

a. They shouldn't gaze at the flickering object such as a candle, b. They should choose a steady object, c. True, d. A & B

Multiple Choice Questions

Q177. Moorchha pranayama is highly advisable for general people suffering from anxiety / mental tension.

a. This is an advanced pranayama, not recommended for a general practitioner, b. True, c. They should do plavini instead., d. Once in a week

Q178. In Ujjayi pranayama, the exhale should be done through-

a. Ida, b. Pingala, c. Both the nostrils, d. Mouth

Q179. Which pranayama helps in curbing hunger and thirst ?

a. Sheetkari, b. Sheetali, c. Anuloma-Viloma, d. A & B

Q180. How many mudras are mentioned in HYP?

a. 6, b. 10, c. 5, d. 8

Q181. Why is Hatha Yoga considered a very practical regimen in modern times?

a. Because it follows a bodily approach, b. Because it works on all 5 parameters of physical fitness, c. Because it lets you move on to the higher spiritual practices while not ignoring the body, d. All of the above

Q182. In Hatha yoga practitioners are supposed to hold a yoga postures with stubborn-ness even if it is hurting them.

a. False, Hatha basically means the balancing of Ha, and Tha (Ida and Pingala) and not only holding the asana, b. True

Q183. Hatha Yoga is best suited for young adults.

a. False, anyone from age of 9 can practice hatha yoga, b. True

Q184. Pregnant women should only practice pranayama and Dhyan. As, Mudra, Bandha and asana can be harmful for the child.

a. False, There are specific mudras, Bandhas and asana for the healthy development of the child., b. True

Q185. Which asana helps in improving the balance?

a. Mayurasana, b. Kukkutasana, b. Matsyendrasana, d. A & B

Q186. Which asana is considered best for Diabetes- '

a. Matsyendrasna, b. Veerasana, c. Mayurasana, d. A & C

Q187. Which practice is beneficial to get rid of Enlargement of the glands?

a. Dhauti, b. Basti, c. Nauli, d. Bhastrika

Q188. Which practice is beneficial to improve the executive functions of the brain?

a. Bhastrika, b. Kapalbhati, c. Anuloma-Viloma, d. Trataka

Q189. What is the average number of breaths per minute?

a. 15, b. 20, c. 12, d.19

Q190. Which practice helps in stimulating the thyroid gland?

a. ujjayi, b. Savasana, c. Suryabhedi, d. Kapalbhati

Q191. tatra pratyayaikatanata_____

a. Dhyanam, b. Dharna, c. Pratyahara, d. None of the above

Q192. Which is part of Purushartha Chatushthya

a. Viveka, b. Vairagya, c. Dharma, d. Sama

Q193. Dharma means-

a. Duty, b. Religion, c. Culture, d. Family values

Q194. Dharma is to be followed by Sanyasins only

a. True, b. False

Q195. Which activities are co-dependent.

a. Artha and Kama, b. Dharma and Kama, c. Moksha and Kama, d. Dharma and Artha

Q196. Which stage of human life is referred to as Vanprastha?

a. 25-50 years, b. 50-75 years, c. 75-100 years, d. 50-65 years

Q197. The meaning of Purusha in the context of purushartha chatushthya is -

a. All males, b. Self, c. Every species on this planet, d. None of the above.

Q198. Kathopnishad is part of which Veda-

a. Krishna Yajurveda, b. Shukla Yajurveda, c. Rigveda, d. Atharvaveda

Q199. As per Kathopnishad, Yoga is-

a. The stillness of the senses, b. Union of Individual self with supreme self, c. Samadhi, d. Dhyana

Q200. Prashnopnishad is part of which Veda?

a. Atharva Veda, b. Rigveda, c. Yajurveda, d. Samaveda

Q201. What is name of the sage who was approched for the questions in Prashnopnishad ?

a. Sage Pipalada, b. Sage Yajnavalkya, c. Sage Nachiketa, d. Sage Ved Vyasa

Q202. "As a king commands his officers, saying to them, Reside in and govern these or those villages, so does this Prana dispose of the other Pranas each for their separate work." This statement is in context of which concept ?

a. Panch Prana, b. Aum, c. Nadis,, d. Atman

Q203. Tattirya Upanishad is part of which Upanishad?

a. Krishna Yajurveda, b. Rigveda, c. Yajurveda, d. Samaveda

Q204. Match the following -

Kathopnishad ---------------Sage Gautama

Tattiryaopnishad------------Nachiketa

Prashnopinishad------------Sage Pipalada

Samkhya---------------------Sage Yajnavalkya

a. a-b, b-d, c-c, d-a, b. a-d, b-b, c-c, d-a, c. a-a, b-b, c-c, d-d, d. a-c, b-a, c-d, d-b

Q205. Which Kosha is made of panch Mahabhutas?

a. Annamaya Kosha, b. Pranamaya Kosha, c. Vijnanamaya Kosha, d. Anandamaya Kosha

Q206. The enquiry into the bliss is referred as-

a. Anand Mimamsa, b. Pancha Kosha Viveka, c. Bhakti, d. Ishwara Pranidhana

Q207. As per Anand Mimamsa, the happiness felt in Brahma Loka (The highest heaven) is the same as-

a. One unit of Human happiness, b. Happiness felt by follower of Veda who is unattached by desires, c. Unparallel to anything, d. None of the above.

Q208. Antahkarna Chatushtaya involves –

a. Chitta, Vritti, Manas, Ahamkara, b. Chitta, Buddhi, Manas, Ahamkara, c. Chitta, Buddhi, Manas, d. Chitta, Buddhi, Anand, Ahamkara

Multiple Choice Questions

Q209. Which of these can be Aklishta Vritti

a. Pratyaksha, b. Viparyaya, c. Smriti, d. All of the above

Q210. Kleshas can be removed by practicing -

a. Surya Namasakar, b. Pratipaksha Bhavna, c. Dhyan Abhyas, d. Yama and Niyama

Q211. False Perception / Illusion is referred to as

a. Avirati, b. Bhranti-Darshan, c. Alabdha - Bhumikatva, d. Anavasthitattva

Q212. The practice of _____ Kumbhak is referred to as eligibility of dharna in PYS.

a. Bahya Kumbhaka, b. Antar Kumbhaka, c. fourth Kumbhaka, d. Bandha with Kumbhaka

Q213. Pramāṇa _____ vikalpa nidrā smṛtayaḥ

a. viparyaya, b. Itaratra, c. Nirodhah, d. None of the above

Q214. Yoga Bhashya is written by

a. Sage Veda Vyasa, b. Sage Patanjali, c. Sage Swatmaram, d. Sage Gheranda

Q215. Which is these is referred as donkey mind?

a. Moodha Chitta, b. Kshipta Chitta, c. Vikshipta Chitta, d. Ekagra Chitta

Multiple Choice Questions

Q216. Tremors in body means-

a. Angamejayatva, b. Svsa-Prasvasa, c. Anavasthitattva, d. None of the above

Q217. Which of these are Pramana Vritti?

a. Pratyaksha, b. Anumana, c. Agama, d. All of the above

Q218. Which asana is considered best as per PYS

a. Padmasana, b. Swastikasana, c. Sukhasana, d. None of the above

Q219. Which one of these are not part of Niyama.

a. Aparigraha, b. Shaucha, c. Santosha, d. Ishwara Pranidhana

Q220. Which one of this is mentioned as pranayama in PYS?

a. Modification of inhalation, b. Suryabhedi, c. Sectional Breathing, d. Ujjayi

Q221. Non-stealing is -

a. Asteya, b. Aparigraha, c. Ishwara Pranidhana, d. Kriya Yoga

Q222. Which is not part of Antaranga Yoga-

a. Pratyharaha, b. Dharna, c. Dhyana, d. Samadhi

Q223. Dhyan is a state of

a. An uninterrupted flow of thoughts toward the object, b. A state of thoughtlessness, c. Withdrawal of senses from the outside world, d. It can not be explained.

Multiple Choice Questions

Q224. Pratyahara is -

a. Concentration, b. Meditation, c. Withdrawal of senses, d. Transcendental stage

Q225. Samadhi means death-

a. True, b. False

Q226. Types of Samadhi as mentioned in PYS

a. Sabija Samadhii, b. Nirbija Samadhi, c. Dharma-Megha samadhi, d. All of the above

Q227. What is the 8th limb of Ashtanga Yoga

a. Dharna, b. Dhyana, c. Samadhi, d. None of the above

Q228. Which Dhyana is considered best as per Gheranda Samhita?

a. Sukshmna Dhyan, b. Sthoola Dhyana, c. Tejo Dhyan, d. Nadanushandhan

Q229. Sagarbha and Nigarbha are types of which pranayama?

a. Sahita, b. Nadi Shodhana, c. Kevali, d. None of the above

Q230. Which one is part of Yama as per HYP?

a. Aparigraha, b. Ishwara Pranidhana, c. Swadhyaya, d. Ahimsa

Q231. Which one is not part of Niyama as per HYP?

a. Tapah, b. Santosh, c. Astikyam, d. Shaucham

Multiple Choice Questions

Q232. Which one is part of Sadhaka Tattva?

a. Atyaharah, b. Prayasa, c. Prajalpo, d. Sahas

Q233. Which one is part of Badhaka Tattva?

a. Tattva-Jnana, b. Nischya, c. Janasangha-Parityaga, d. Lolyam

Q234. Hri means-

a. Modesty, b. Discerning intellect, c. Mantra repetition, d. Sacrifice

Q235. Prajalpa Means-

a. Over-exertion, b. Talkativeness, c. Over-adhering to the rules, d. Perseverance

Q236. Panchadharana (as per GS) includes-

a. Prithvi (earth), b. Ambhasi (water), c. Vayavi (Aerial), d. All of the above

Q237. How many types of Samadhi are mentioned in GS?

a. 1, b. 2, c. 4, d. 6

Q238. On average, human beings breathe almost-

a. 21600 in 24 hours, b. 20000 in 24 hours, c. 18000 in 24 hours, d. None of the above

Q239. Respiration refers to -

a. The exchange of oxygen and carbon-di-oxide, b. Inhale and exhale, c. A&B both, d. None of the above

Q240. What should be the length of the Hermitage of the yogi?

a. 1 mtr, b. 1.5 meter, c. 3 meter, d. None of the above

Q241. Nadi is a complex mechanism that allows the flow of -

a. Prana, b. Blood, c. Lipid, d. Water

Q242. Nadis originates from -

a. Brahmarandha, b. Shikha Mandal, c. Visshudhu Chakra, d. Kandasthan

Q243. As per Shiva Samhita, how many nadis are there?

a. 350,000, b. 300,000, c. 72,000, d. 3

Q244. Which Nadi is linked to the parasympathetic nervous system?

a. Ida, b. Pingala, c. Susumna, d. None of the above

Q245. Which Nadi is linked to the sympathetic nervous system?

a. Ida, b. Pingala, c. Susumna, d. None of the above

Q246. The different layers of Susumna are-

a. Vajra, b. Chitrani, c. Brahma, d. All of the above

Q247. When Ida Nadi is activated one should do the-

a. The Tasks that require mental creativity, b. The task which requires thinking and planning c. None of the above, d. All of the above

Multiple Choice Questions

Q248. When Pingala Nadi is activated one should do the-

a. The tasks that require physical activity, b. The task which requires execution, c. None of the above, d. A&B Both

Q249. The breath alternates between Ida and Pingala every-

a. 60-90 minutes, b. 60-120 minutes, c. 23-48 hours, d. 24 hours

Q250. Kumbhaka refers to -

a. Retention, b. To inhale, c. To exhale, d. To hold

Q251. The basic difference between Ashtanga Yoga and Hatha Yoga can be understood as

a. Ashtanga Yoga is a mind-oriented approach whereas Hatha Yoga is a body-oriented approach,b.In Hatha Yoga Body is used as a medium to eventually achieve the Raja Yoga. In Ashtanga Yoga, Mind is used as a medium to achieve the Raja Yoga,c.Both lineages follow the same approaches,d.A & B

Q252. Which practice is suggested by Patanjali, in combination with Vairagaya to achieve mental balance.

a. Abhyasa, b. Ashtanga Yoga, c. Pratipaksha Bhavana, d. Ishvara Pranidhana

Q253. "A feeling of anger towards someone should immediately be replaced by the feeling of love" This practice is known by –

a. Chitta Prasadanam, b. Pratipaksha Bhavna, c. Santosha, d. Aparigraha

Q254. One should keep an attitude of mudita (cheerfulness) towards-

a. Happy people, b. Virtuous People, c. Artharthi, d. Jigyasu

Q255. It is suggested in Yoga Sutra to keep the bhava of upekshanam (Avoidance / Indifference) towards people who are evil.

a. True, b. False

Q256. Patanjali suggests practicing multiple techniques as per the situations to achieve mental balance.

a. False, Patanjali suggests to practice Ektattva Abhayas (Practicing one technique) to achieve highest mental wellbeing, b. True

Q257. The practice of non possessiveness is part of-

a. Yama, b. Niyama, c. Kriya Yoga, d. Eka Tatva Abhyasa

Q258. The antaryas mentioned in Yoga Sutra can be understood as fundamental causes of mental illness and Sahbhuvas can be understood as the consequences.

a. True, b. False

Multiple Choice Questions

Q259. Styan is one of the Anatrayas, which means-

a. , b. Unable to attain stability, c. Unable to maintain stability, d. Mental Lethargy

Q260. Daur Manasya is one of the Sahabhuvas which means-

a. Depression, b. Distress, c. Eustress, d. ADHD

Q261. Pratyahara is referred to as the bridge between Bahiranga yoga and Antaranga Yoga because-

a. It prepares the mind for Meditation, b. The meditation is only possible when the senses are withdrawn from the outside stimuli, c. Before Pratyahara, all the practices were possible due to sense involvement, In Pratyahara, a senseless perception is practiced, d. All of the above

Q262. The eligibility of Dharna is -

a. Pratyahara, b. Pranayama, c. Asana, d. Practice

Q263. Meditation (Dhyana) can be understood as a result of consistent practice of Concentration (Dharana).

a. True, b. False

Q264. Samadhi can be understood as a result of the consistent practice of Dhyana.

a. True, b. False

Q265. Which limb is referred to as social constraints-

a. Yama, b. Niyama, c. Abhyasa, d. Klesha

Q266. Ahimsa (Non-violence) is the practice of-

a. Keeping violent thoughts away from the mind, b. Staying away from the violent actions, c. Not involved in the violent conversation, d. All of the above

Q267. The practice of Saucha is -

a. Cleanliness of thoughts, body, surroundings, etc., b. Cleanliness of body only, c. Cleanliness of toilet, d. Cleanliness of house

Q268. Contentment should be practiced all the time irrespective of the situation one is in.

a. True, b. False

Q269. Ishwara Pranidhana is a practice of surrendering to -

a. Personal God, b. A supreme power, c. Self, d. Nature

Q270. Dharana, Dhyana, and Samadhi; collectively is a step-by-step process and when it happens together it is referred to as -

a. Nirbija Samadhi, b. Sabija Samadhi, c. Samyama, d. Dharma Megha Samadhi

Q271. As per the Bhagavad Gita, how many qualities are mentioned as divine virtues?

a. 24, b. 26, c. 18, d. 16

Multiple Choice Questions

Q272. Which of these is mentioned as one of the saintly virtues?

a. Jnana Yoga, b. Hatha Yoga, c. Vinyasa Yoga, d. Bhakti Yoga

Q273. Dhritih means-

a. Fortitude, b. Gratitude, c. Modesty, d. None of the above

Q274. Bhagavad Gita propounds moderation as the means to mitigate sorrow. Which of these Shloka propounds this concept?

a. 2.48, b. 2.50, c. 6.17, d. 6.19

Q275. Achapalam is the opposite of -

a. Laulyam, b. Aloluptvam, c. Arjavam, d. None of the above

Q276. Fault finding is considered one of the

a. Normal human behavior, b. Saintly virtues, c. Demonic virtue, d. None of the above

Q277. Swadhyaya can be considered as -

a. Study of scriptures, b. Study of the self, c. Study of the supreme, d. A & B

Q278. Arjavam means-

a. Being straightforward, b. Being assertive, c. Being Arrogant, d. A & B

Q279. Qualities like arjavam, akrodha, ati manita can help in setting healthy boundaries to keep mental peace.

a. True, b. False

Q280. Tapah refers to -

a. Secluded practices in the forest, b. Austerities, c. Giving up the worldly life, d. A & B

Q281. What would you suggest to someone with a frozen shoulder?

a. Skandha Sanchalana, b. Gomukhasana, c. Physiotherapy, d. Garudasana

Q282. The person in Depression should be given

a. Pranayama, b. Surya Namaskar, c. Meditation, d. A & B

Q283. The instant relaxation practice would be

a. Yogic Breath, b. Yoga Nidra, c. Bhramari, d. All of the above

Q284. Karma yoga is -

a. Selfless service, b. Detachment from the action, c. Skill in action, d. All of the above

Q285. Someone with a sluggish digestion should practice-

a. Dhauti, b. Basti, c. Neti, d. A & B

Multiple Choice Questions

Q286. Eye fatigue can be prevented/controlled with -

a. Trataka, b. Washing the eyes with water, c. Yoga Nidra, d. Shavasana

Q287. Yoga is a lifestyle based on oneness. It teaches you proper behavior with others as well as with yourself. Which practices are in support of this statement?

a. Yama & Niyama, b. Chaturanga Yoga, c. Asana & Pranyama, d. Abhyasa and Vairgya

Q288. The fundamental cause of illness is an imbalance of doshas. There are yogic practices to balance the doshas and achieve optimum health. Which practices are in support of this statement?

a. Shatkarma, b. Pranayama, c. Mudra, d. All of the above

Q289. Which practices should be followed to control anxiety and panic attacks?

a. Yogic Deep Breathing, b. Anuloma Viloma, c. Chest opening and Spine stretching asanas, d. All of the above

Q290. Which practices should be followed to boost the contentment within oneself?

a. Self Analysis, b. Accepting oneself, c. Karma Yoga, d. All of the above

Q291. The powerhouse of the cell is called as-

a. Organelles, b. Mitochondria, c. Cytoplasm, d. Cell wall

Q292. The largest bone in the body is -

a. Tibia, b. Fibula, c. Femur, d. Spine

Q293. The total number of bones in the vertebrae column is-

a. 26, b. 34, c. 35, d. 36

Q294. Which one of these is the hip bone?

a. Sacrum, b. Ilium, c. Carpal, d. Phalanges

Q295. The structure which attaches muscle to a bone is called-

a. Tendon, b. Ligament, c. Joint, d. Fascia

Q296. What is also called a voice box?

a. Pharynx, b. Larynx, c. Tonsils, d. Trachea

Q297. What is the function of the artery

a. To transport the oxygen-rich blood from the heart to the body, b. To transport the oxygen-blood from the body to the heart, c. To participate in gas exchange, d. None of the above

Multiple Choice Questions

Q298. What is the function of the Pulmonary Artery?

a. To transport the oxygen-poor blood from the heart to the lungs, b. To transport the oxygen-rich blood from the lungs to the heart, c. To act as a parent artery which helps in supplying oxygen-rich blood to the other arteries and then to the body, d. B & C

Q299. What is a coronary circuit?

a. A channel that provides blood to the heart, b. A channel that provides between the heart and lungs, c. A channel that provides blood for the Corona patient, d. None of the above

Q300. Which part of the brain is also known as the "center of respiration"

a. Cerebrum, b. Hypothalamus, c. Medulla Oblongata, d. Midbrain

Q301. The oxygen rich blood get pumped into the body from heart through-

a. Aorta, b. Superior Vena Cava, c. Capillaries, d. Arteriole Capillaries

Q302. What is the pH level of pure water?

a. 6.1, b. 7, c. 8.2, d. 6.4

Q303. Which system triggers the Fight / Flight response?

a. Sympathetic Nervous System, b. Parasympathetic Nervous System, c. Autonomic Nervous System, d. Central Nervous System

Multiple Choice Questions

Q304. The action of swallowing food is known as-

a. Propulsion, b. Ingestion, c. Eating, d. Absorption

Q305. Which organ is not the part of Digestive System-

a. Pancreas, b. Liver, c. Large Intestine, d. Kidney

Q306. The example of ductless glands is -

a. Sebaceous, b. Mammary Gland, c. Parathyroid Gland, d. None of the above

Q307. What is the major role of calcium in the body?

a. To provide the electrical energy for nervous and muscular system, b. To strengthen the bones, c. To help in growing, d. To help in thyroid gland's health

Q308. The prime hormones released by Adrenal Glands are-

a. Epinephrine (Adrenaline), b. Non-Epinephrine (nor-adrenaline), c. Cortisol, d. All of the above

Q309. Which organ has exocrine and endocrine both functionalities?

a. Adrenal, b. Parathyroid, c. Pancreas, d. Gonads

Q310. Islets of Langerhans is -

a. Endocrine part of Pancreas, b. Exocrine part of Pancreas, c. Part of Adrenal Medulla, d. Part of Hypothalamus

Q311. As per PYS, one should aspire to have an attitude of friendship towards people who are -

a. Happy, b. Virtuous, c. Kind, d. Warrior

Q312. The attitude of indifference (Upekshanam) helps you set healthy boundaries-

a. True, b. False

Q313. Mudita means-

a. Cheerfulness, b. Kindness, c. Balanced, d. Neutral

Q314. A group of organs that work together to carry out a particular function, is referred as-

a. Organism, b. Organ System, c. Cell, d. Tissue

Q315. The prime hormone secreted by Testicles is-

a. Growth hormone. b. Testosterone, c. Estrogen, d. Estradiol

Q316. Which hormone is crucial for female growth such as breast development, fallopian tube development, uterus development, etc?

a. Estrogen, b. Estradiol, c. Estriol, d. All of the above

Q317. The liver can store glycogen up to

a. 5% of its mass, b. 10% of its mass, c. 7% of its mass, d. As much as it can hold.

Q318. Whenever there is a rise in the blood sugar level, Pancreas releases-

a. Insulin, b. Glucagon, c. Glycogen, d. Epinephrine

Q319. Which hormone prevents blood glucose levels from dropping too low.

a. Insulin, b. Glucagon, c. Glycogen, d. Epinephrine

Q320. The lymphatic system is part of -

a. Cardiovascular system, b. Circulatory System, c. Nervous system, d. A & C

Q321. How many Bhavas are there?

a. 7, b. 8, c. 6, d. Unlimited

Q322. One of the reasons why yoga practice should be done with mindfulness is because it intensifies the current bhava.

a. True, b. False

Q323. Match the following-

Dharma —Wisdom

Jnana –Strength

Vairagya —Detachment

Aishwarya —Virtue

a. a-d, b-a, c-c, d-b. b. a-d, b-a, c-b, d-c, c. a-a, b-b, c-c, d-b, d. a-c, b-d, c-a, d-b

Multiple Choice Questions

Q324. Match the following-

Adharma — Ignorance

Ajnana —Vice

Raga —Weakness

An-Aishwarya —Attachment

a. a-b, b-a, c-d, d-c, b. a-c, b-a, c-d, d-b, c. a-b, b-c, c-d, d-a, d. a-b, b-a, c-c, d-d

Q325. Discipline is another aspect of –?

a. Aishwarya, b. Jnana, c. Dharma, d. Vairagya

Q326. Twisting, lateral and upward postures help in strengthening which Bhava?

a. Dharma, b. Jnana, c. Vairagya, d. Aishwarya

Q327. Forward bendings help in strengthening which Bhava?

a. Vairagya, b. Jnana, c. Dharma, d. Raga

Q328. Ajnana means - ?

a. Devoid of knowledge, b. Knowing the opposite of the truth, c. External knowledge, d. Not knowing the scriptures

Q329. Abhyasa_____ tan nirodhah?

a. Vairagyabhyam, b. Vairagya, c. Vairagi, d. Chittah

Q330. How many Kleshas are there?

a. 5, b. 4, c. 9, d. 6

Multiple Choice Questions

Q331. Nasya is -

a. Putting oil in nose, b. Oil pulling, c. Jala Neti, d. Blowing the nose first thing in the morning

Q332. Kshaura Karma is -

a. Defecation and urination, b. Regular cutting of hair, nails, etc, c. Deodorants, perfumes, face-pack, etc, d. Body massage with oil

Q333. Which kriya helps in ensuring mouth health?

a. Oil Pulling, b. Gargling, c. Smoke inhaling, d. Herbs chewing

Q334. As per Ayurveda Vata is dominating between-

a. 6 AM – 10 AM and 6 PM – 10 PM, b. 2 AM – 6 AM and 2 PM – 6 PM, c. 10 AM – 2 PM and 10 PM – 2 AM, d. None of the above

Q335. The best time to eat the largest meal of the day is -

a. Pitta dominating 10 Am -2 PM, b. Vata dominating- 2 PM - 6 PM, c. Pitta dominating- 6 AM to 10 AM, d. Kapha dominating- 6 PM to 10 PM

Q336. Vasant Ritu (Spring) occurs -

a. Mid-March to Mid-May, b. Mid-May to Mid-July, c. Mid- Jan to Mid-March, d. Mid-July to Mid-September

Multiple Choice Questions

Q337. Vata dosha aggravates during which season?

a. Sharad Ritu, b. Vasant Ritu, c. Varsha Ritu, d. Grishma Ritu

Q338. Pitta Auto-pacifies during which season?

a. Hemant Ritu, b. Varsha Ritu, c. Grishma Ritu, d. Sharad Ritu

Q339. How many kaals are there in a year?

a. 12, b. 6, c. 2, d. 3

Q340. Dinacharya and Ritucharya is for -

a. Males, b. Grihastha, c. Vidyarthi, d. All of the above

Q341. A disease is -

a. Particular abnormal condition, b. One of the 9 antaryas, c. Signs that something is wrong with the body, d. All of the above

Q342. Patanjali says Vyadhi (Disease) usually accompany the -

a. Sahabhuvas, b. Fluctuation in mind, c. Weakness, d. Kleshas

Q343. Adhi can be understood as-

a. Physical disease, b. Disturbed mind, c. Disease, d. A & B

Multiple Choice Questions

Q344. Angamejaytava is -

a. Irregular breathing flow, b. Tremors in the body, c. Unhappiness, d. Depression

Q345. Heyam Dukham Anagatam means-

a. Prevention of the future pain and suffering, b. Treatment of the disease, c. Pain management, d. None of the above

Q346. Yoga is a wonderful preventive care.

a. True as there are different practices which target different areas. Such as Shat kriyas for internal cleansing, Asana for body strength, Pranayama for breath control etc. b. False, Medicines are the only way to live healthy.

Q347. Yoga is called holistic as it focuses on all the aspects of health, even spiritual.

a. True, the attitude of Ishwar Pranidhana leads to spiritual awareness, b. False, Yoga considers many health aspect but not all, such as weight loss.

Q348. The moral values can be inculcated by practicing-

a. Yama, b. Ishvara Pranidhana, c. Chitta Prasadana, d. Kriya Yoga

Q349. How many bones are there in the human body ?

a. 206, b. 106, c. 600, d. 202

Multiple Choice Questions

Q350. Red bone marrow is produced at-

a. Vertebrae, b. Breastbone, c. Pelvis, d. All of the above

Q351. CPR stands for?

a. Cardiopulmonary Resuscitation, b. Californians for Pesticide Reform, c. Computerized Patient Record, d. Command Performance Review

Q352. First aid refers to -

a. Immediate medical attention to the injury, b. Medical attention after 15 minutes of threat, c. Medical attention is given only by the doctors, d. None of the above

Q353. What is CPR?

a. An emergency lifesaving procedure, b. An emergency first aid, c. A procedure which happens in the ICU, d. A treatment for the pulmonary issues

Q354. Immediate CPR can double or triple the chances of survival after cardiac arrest.

a. True, b. False

Q355. What is the compressions-to-breaths ratio in CPR?

a. 30:2, b. 30:5, c. 25:2, d. 25:5

Q356. While giving compressions, how much depth should be maintained?

a. 2-2.4 inches, b. 3 inches, c. 5 inches, d. 1 inch

Multiple Choice Questions

Q357. What is hand only CPR?

a. A technique for untrained people to only give compressions, b. Compressions without mouth to mouth breath, c. A technique which uses no compressions, d. A & B

Q358. Drinking fluids to relieve heat stress, is part of -

a. First Aid, b. CPR, c. Ambulance treatment, d. Recovery treatment

Q359. Which is the smallest bone in the body ?

a. Stapes, b. Patella, c. Phalanges, d Knuckles

Q360. Ribs that are directly attached to the sternum via costal cartilages are called-

a. True ribs, b. False ribs, c. Floating ribs, d. None of the above

Q361. The process by which the body converts whatever we eat and drink into energy is called -

a. Digestion, b. Absorption, c. Anabolism, d. None of the above

Q362. A result of the pathological response of the body to either external or internal factors is referred as-

a. Disease, b. Disorder, c. Syndrome, d. Condition

Q363. Disruption of the usual bodily functions due to the presence of disease in the body is referred to as -

a. Disorder, b. Syndrome, c. Condition, d. None of the above

Q364. An abnormal state that feels different from your normal state of well-being is referred to as

a. Disease, b. Disorder, c. Syndrome, d. Condition

Q365. When an abnormal chemical reaction in the body disrupts the usual energy conversion process, is referred to as -

a. Diabetes, b. Metabolic disorder, c. Low sugar level, d. Thyroidism

Q366. The keys factor to managing Metabolic disorders is -

a. Right Food, b. Physical Activity, c. Proper sleep, d. All of the above

Q367. For asthma patients which asanas are beneficial?

a. Padahastasana, b. Katichakrasana, c. Balasana, d. A & C

Q368. Which asanas are beneficial for Diabetic patients?

a. Matsyendrasana, b. Dhanurasana, c. Paschimottanasana, d. All of the above

Q369. FVC stands for -

a. Forced Ventilation Capacity, b. Forced Vital Capacity, c. Frequent Vital Capacity, d. A & B

Q370. The ribs which don't attach to the sternum at all are called -

a. Floating Ribs, b. False Ribs, c. True Ribs, d. None of the above

Q371. Personality can be defined as -

a. Characteristic patterns of thoughts, feelings and behaviors that make a person unique, b. A combination of traits and patterns that influence behavior, thought motivation, and emotion, c. A characteristic way of thinking, feeling, and behaving, d. All of the above

Q372. Which practices help in developing social values?

a. Principles of Yama, b. Asana, c. Kriya Yoga, d. Chitta Prasadana

Q373. Which practices work on the emotional dimension of personality?

a. Dhyana, b. Trataka, c. Pranayama, d. All of the above

Q374. Yogic practices should be introduced as early as 8 years for an holistic development of the child.

a. True, b. False

Q375. Human skeleton is divided into -

a. Axial Skeleton and Appendicular Skeleton, b. Axial Skeleton and Vertebrae columns, c. Bones and muscles, d. Upper limbs and lower limbs

Multiple Choice Questions

Q376. Tissues which connect 2 muscles are called-

a. Fascia, b. Ligament, c. Tendon, d. Connective tissues

Q377. The joints which are found between the bones of the skull are called-

a. Gomphosis, b. Syndesmosis, c. Suture, d. Fibrous Joint

Q378. Wrist is an example of -

a. Saddle Joint, b. Condyloid Joint, c. Pivot Joint, d. Plane / Gliding Joint

Q379. What is the basic unit of the nervous system?

a. Neuron, b. Nephron, c. Mitochondria, d. Nerves

Q380. What is the basic unit of kidney function?

a. Nephrons, b. Neurons, c. Cells, d. RBC

Q381. The light signal is converted into electrical impulses by

a. Retina, b. Optic Nerve, c. Pupil, d. None of the above

Q382. The colored portion of the eye is -

a. Iris, b. Lens, c. Pupil, d. Cornea

Q383. Which cells are responsible for vision in low light-

a. Rods, b. Cones, c. Corena, d. Lens

Multiple Choice Questions

Q384. The olfactory cortex is responsible for -

a. Sense of smell, b. Sense of touch, c. Sense of vision, d. Sense of taste

Q385. The rough texture of the tongue is because of -

a. Papillae, b. Mucosa, c. Lymph Nodes, d. None of the above

Q386. The term Ossicles collectively refers to -

a. Malleus, Incus, and Stapes, b. Mucous Gland, Serous Gland, and Lymph nodes, c. Superior Semicircular Canal, Posterior Semicircular Canal, and Lateral Semicircular Canal, d. None of the above

Q387. The system which forms the outermost layer of the body is called-

a. Integumentary system, b. Merkel cells system, c. Cochlea, d. External Meatus

Q388. Skin is the site for Vitamin D synthesis.

a. True, b. False

Q389. Which is the largest organ in the body?

a. Liver, b. Skin, c. Small Intestine, d. Large Intestine.

Q390. The sound waves are converted into electrical impulses by

a. Cochlea, b. Eardrum, c. Stapes, d. Incus

Multiple Choice Questions

Q391. What is the pH level of blood?

a. 7.35 to 7.45, b. 4.5, c. 7.10, d. 8

Q392. What should be the pH level of the drinking water?

a. 6.5–8.5, b. 5.5- 5.6, c. 4.6-4.8, d. None of the above

Q393. The process of maintaining a stable state within the body is referred as-

a. Homeostasis, b. Photosynthesis, c. The negative feedback loop, d. None of the above

Q394. What are the processes that are maintained through Homeostasis?

a. The water level in the body, b. The temperature of the body, c. Production of the sound, d. A&B both

Q395. Segmentation occurs in -

a. Esophagus, b. Large Intestine, c. Mouth, d. Stomach

Q396. The curled part of the small intestine is called-

a. Jejunum, b. Duodenum, c. ileum, d. Colon

Q397. The basic function kidney is -

a. Filter waste from the blood, b. sweating, c. Controlling body chemistry, d. A&B Both

Q398. Peptide hormones are-

a. Lipophobic, b. Lipophilic, c. Hydrophilic, d. A&C both

Multiple Choice Questions

Q399. The hormone responsible to prevent blood glucose levels from dropping too low is -

a. Insulin, b. Glucagon, c. Glycogen, d. Trypsin

Q400. The main sites where Glycogen is stored are-

a. Liver and Adipose tissues, b. Pancreas, c. The small intestine, d. Bones

Q401. Nasal Irrigation refers to -

a. Oil pulling, b. Jala Neti, c. Blowing the nose first thing in the morning, d. None of the above

Q402. Abhyanga is -

a. Defecation and urination, b. Regular cutting of hair, nails, etc, c. Deodorants, perfumes, face-pack, etc, d. Body massage with oil

Q403. Dhooma pana is ?

a. Oil Pulling, b. Gargling, c. Medicated Smoke inhaling, d. Herbs chewing

Q404. Autumn occurs -

a. Mid-Sep to Mid-Nov, b. Mid-May to Mid-July, c. Mid-Jan to Mid-March, d. Mid-July to Mid-September

Q405. Dinacharya refers to -

a. Daily activity, b. Seasonal activity, c. Weekly activity, d. None of the above

Multiple Choice Questions

Q406. Match the following -

Shishira - astringent

Vasanata- sour

Greeshma - bitter

Varsha - pungent

a. A-C, B-A, C-D, D- B, b. A-B, B-A, C-D, D- C, c. A-C, B-A, C-B, D- D, d. A-C, B-D, C-B, D- A

Q407. Which dosha accumulates in Winter and aggravates in Spring

a. Kapha, b. Vata, c. Pitta, d. A&C

Q408. Abhyanga should be done immediately after attending to natural urges (malotsarga).

a. True, b. False

Q409. Pitta dohsa aggravates in which season?

a. Autumn, b. Winter, c. Spring, d. Summer

Q410. Hemanta ritu occurs-

a. Mid-November to Mid-January, b. Mid-January to Mid-March, c. Mid-September to Mid-November, d. None of the above

Q411. Tridosha refers to

a. Vata, Pitta, Kapha, b. Agni, Vayu, Mala, c. Satva, Rajas, and Tamas, d. None of the above

Q412. When Pitta abnormally decreases-

a. Gastric fire will be reduced, b. loss of sensation will occur, c. Dizziness will occur, d. All of the above

Q413. Kapha is at its peak during -

a. Brahma Muhurta, b. Morning and evening, c. Late night, d. None of the above

Q414. Which Vayu is responsible for digestion -

a. Prana, b. Udana, c. Samana, d. Apana

Q415. Which pitta is responsible for the luster of the skin?

a. Pachaka Pitta, b. Ranjaka Pitta, c. Bhrajaka Pitta, d. Alochaka Pitta

Q416. Which Kapha has the binding property?

a. Sleshka Kapha, b. Kledaka Kapha, c. Tarpaka Kapha, d. Avalambaka Kapha

Q417. Which one is not a Dhatu?

a. Rasa, b. Meda, c. Sukra, d. Agni

Q418. Agni is of -

a. 13 types, b. 15 types, c. 20 types, d. Only one fire

Q419. Which is, not a mala?

a. Pureesha, b. Mootra, c. Sveda, d. Sukra

Multiple Choice Questions

Q420. Vata auto-pacifies in -

a. Autumn (Sharad Ritu), b. Summer (Grishma Ritu), c. The rainy season (Varsha Ritu), d. Winter (Hemant Ritu)

Q421. Trayopstambha includes-

a. Ahara, b. Nidra, c. Dhyana, d. A & B

Q422. Proper diet, digestion, and elimination are paramount to our well-being.

a. True, b. False

Q423. The vital energy that protects the body and mind from disease and gives us great vigor and longevity

a. Ojas, b. Rajas, c. Sattva, d. All of the above

Q424. Charak Samhita is written by -

a. Maharishi Charaka, b. Maharishi Sushuruta, c. Maharishi Patanjali, d. Maharishi Veda Vyasa

Q425. The way we engage in action is as impactful as the action itself.

a. True, b. False, c. Not Sure

Q426. When_____is depleted, Ojas is Depleted.

a. Blood, b. Shukra, c. Meda, d. Rasa

Q427. The best time to wake up as per Ayurveda is-

a. Brahma muhurta, b. As per your situation, c. After Sunrise, d. None of the above

Multiple Choice Questions

Q428. Being lethargic, stagnant, and excessively sleepy is a sign of -

a. Imabalnce in kapha, b. Imbalance in Vata, c. Imbalance in Pitta, d. All of the above

Q429. To ensure that the food works best for our body, we should ensure-

a. Proper combination, b. Proper timing, c. Mindful eating, d. All of the above

Q430. As per Ayurveda, one should not indulge in sexual activity at all.

a. True, b. False

Q431. Which practice should be part of Acidity Management?

a. Agnisar Kriya, b. Kohni Naman, c. Sarvangasana, d. Shavasana

Q432. IBS is a condition of-

a. Inflamed colon, b. Loosen sphincter muscles of the esophagus, c. Inflamed lungs, d. None of the above

Q433. Vastra Dhauti is effective in -

a. Constipation, Indigestion, Bloating, b. High Blood pressure, Low Blood pressure, c. Depression, Anxiety, Tensional Headache, d. All of the above

Q434. The instrument to measure BP is called-

a. Sphygmomanometer, b. Stethoscope, c. Ophthalmoscope, d. Defibrillator

Multiple Choice Questions

Q435. The contraindicatory practice for HBP is

a. Vipreetkarni, b. Bhastrika, c. Bahya Kumbhaka, d. All of the above

Q436. The contraindicatory practice for Cervical Spondylosis is -

a. Sarvangasana, Setu- bandh asana, and Halasana, b. Chin locking, Jalandhara Bandha,, c. Ujjayi, d. All of the above

Q437. Which practices should be part of lower back management?

a. Bhujangasna, Shalabhasana, b. Supta Udarakarshanasana, Ardha Chakrasana, c. Paschimottasana, Janu Sheershasana, d. A & B

Q438. Type 2 Diabetese is -

a. Metabolic Disorder, b. Genetic Disorder, c. Lifestyle Disorder, d. A & C

Q439. The largest amount of air that a person can inhale and then exhale during a 12- to 15-s interval with maximal voluntary effort is known as

a. MVV, b. PEFR, c. FVC, d. Respiration

Q440. The maximal volume of air that can be exhaled after maximum inhalation is referred as-

a. Vital Capacity, b. Total Lung Capacity, c. Lung Volume, d. None of the above

Multiple Choice Questions

Q441. International Yoga Day is celebrated on?

a. 21st June, b. 26th June, c. 21st May, d. 22nd June

Q442. The theme of the first International Yoga Day was-

a. Yoga for Harmony & Peace, b. Yoga for heath, c. Yoga for peace, d. Yoga for heart

Q443. The first International Yoga Day was celebrated in-

a. New Delhi, b. Lucknow, c. Dehradun, d. Ranchi

Q444. What is the theme of International Day of Yoga 2021?

a. Yoga for wellness, b. Yoga for all, c. Yoga for people, d. None of the above.

Q445. What is the theme of International Day of Yoga 2020?

a. Climate change, b. Yoga for health- Yoga at home, c. Connect the youth, d. Yoga for health

Q446. What is the name of the video blogging contest jointly organized by the Ministry Of Ayush (MOA) and the Indian Council Of Cultural Relations (ICCR) in 2020?

a. My words and yoga, b. Practicing yoga, c. My life, my yoga, d. Yoga is life.

Q447. What was the theme for International Day of Yoga 2023?

a. Yoga for peace, b. Yoga for all, c. Yoga for Vasudheva Kutumbkam, d. Yoga for unity

Q448. Mental hygiene can be brought in by practicing

a. Meditation, b. Charity, c. Yama & Niyama, d. None of the above.

Q449. According to Patanjali..........can lead to perfection in the state of Samadhi

a. Ahimsa, b. Aparigraha, c. Ishwara Pranidhan, d. Pratipaksha Bhawana

Q450. Which sense organ represents Space?

a. Tongue, b. Ear, c. Eye, d. Skin

ANSWERS

Q1	a	Q28	b	Q55	b	Q82	c	Q109	b
Q2	a	Q29	b	Q56	a	Q83	b	Q110	a
Q3	b	Q30	d	Q57	d	Q84	d	Q111	a
Q4	b	Q31	a	Q58	c	Q85	d	Q112	a
Q5	a	Q32	a	Q59	a	Q86	b	Q113	b
Q6	a	Q33	a	Q60	a	Q87	b	Q114	a
Q7	a	Q34	a	Q61	c	Q88	b	Q115	b
Q8	a	Q35	a	Q62	a	Q89	a	Q116	a
Q9	a	Q36	a	Q63	d	Q90	a	Q117	a
Q10	b	Q37	a	Q64	a	Q91	b	Q118	a
Q11	a	Q38	b	Q65	c	Q92	c	Q119	a
Q12	d	Q39	a	Q66	a	Q93	a	Q120	b
Q13	b	Q40	a	Q67	d	Q94	a	Q121	b
Q14	b	Q41	b	Q68	b	Q95	a	Q122	a
Q15	c	Q42	b	Q69	a	Q96	a	Q123	a
Q16	b	Q43	a	Q70	a	Q97	a	Q124	d
Q17	a	Q44	d	Q71	a	Q98	a	Q125	d
Q18	a	Q45	a	Q72	b	Q99	a	Q126	a
Q19	a	Q46	a	Q73	b	Q100	a	Q127	a
Q20	b	Q47	d	Q74	d	Q101	a	Q128	b
Q21	b	Q48	a	Q75	b	Q102	d	Q129	d

Answers

Q22	a	Q49	c	Q76	a	Q103	b	Q130	d
Q23	a	Q50	a	Q77	b	Q104	a	Q131	a
Q24	a	Q51	a	Q78	a	Q105	a	Q132	b
Q25	a	Q52	b	Q79	d	Q106	a	Q133	b
Q26	a	Q53	c	Q80	b	Q107	b	Q134	a
Q27	a	Q54	a	Q81	b	Q108	a	Q135	c

Q136	a	Q163	b	Q190	a	Q217	d
Q137	b	Q164	b	Q191	a	Q218	d
Q138	b	Q165	a	Q192	c	Q219	a
Q139	d	Q166	b	Q193	a	Q220	a
Q140	d	Q167	b	Q194	b	Q221	a
Q141	b	Q168	b	Q195	a	Q222	a
Q142	a	Q169	a	Q196	b	Q223	a
Q143	a	Q170	b	Q197	b	Q224	c
Q144	a	Q171	a	Q198	a	Q225	b
Q145	a	Q172	b	Q199	a	Q226	d
Q146	a	Q173	d	Q200	a	Q227	c
Q147	a	Q174	b	Q201	a	Q228	a
Q148	b	Q175	a	Q202	a	Q229	a
Q149	a	Q176	d	Q203	a	Q230	d
Q150	a	Q177	a	Q204	a	Q231	d
Q151	a	Q178	a	Q205	a	Q232	d
Q152	a	Q179	d	Q206	a	Q233	d
Q153	a	Q180	b	Q207	b	Q234	a
Q154	a	Q181	d	Q208	b	Q235	b
Q155	b	Q182	a	Q209	d	Q236	d
Q156	a	Q183	a	Q210	c	Q237	d
Q157	a	Q184	a	Q211	b	Q238	a
Q158	a	Q185	d	Q212	c	Q239	c

Answers

Q159	b	Q186	a	Q213	a	Q240	b
Q160	a	Q187	b	Q214	a	Q241	a
Q161	a	Q188	b	Q215	a	Q242	d
Q162	c	Q189	a	Q216	a	Q243	a

Q244	a	Q271	b	Q298	a	Q325	c
Q245	b	Q272	a	Q299	a	Q326	b
Q246	d	Q273	a	Q300	c	Q327	a
Q247	d	Q274	c	Q301	a	Q328	b
Q248	d	Q275	a	Q302	b	Q329	a
Q249	a	Q276	c	Q303	a	Q330	a
Q250	a	Q277	d	Q304	a	Q331	a
Q251	d	Q278	d	Q305	d	Q332	b
Q252	a	Q279	a	Q306	c	Q333	a
Q253	b	Q280	d	Q307	a	Q334	b
Q254	b	Q281	a	Q308	d	Q335	a
Q255	a	Q282	d	Q309	c	Q336	a
Q256	a	Q283	d	Q310	a	Q337	c
Q257	a	Q284	d	Q311	a	Q338	a
Q258	a	Q285	d	Q312	a	Q339	c
Q259	d	Q286	a	Q313	a	Q340	d
Q260	a	Q287	a	Q314	b	Q341	d
Q261	d	Q288	d	Q315	b	Q342	a
Q262	b	Q289	d	Q316	b	Q343	b
Q263	a	Q290	d	Q317	a	Q344	b
Q264	a	Q291	b	Q318	a	Q345	a
Q265	a	Q292	c	Q319	b	Q346	a
Q266	d	Q293	a	Q320	b	Q347	a
Q267	a	Q294	b	Q321	b	Q348	a
Q268	a	Q295	a	Q322	a	Q349	a

Answers

Q269	b	Q296	b	Q323	a	Q350	d
Q270	c	Q297	a	Q324	a	Q351	a

Q352	a	Q379	a	Q406	a	Q433	a
Q353	a	Q380	a	Q407	a	Q434	a
Q354	a	Q381	a	Q408	b	Q435	d
Q355	a	Q382	a	Q409	a	Q436	d
Q356	a	Q383	a	Q410	a	Q437	d
Q357	d	Q384	a	Q411	a	Q438	d
Q358	a	Q385	a	Q412	a	Q439	a
Q359	a	Q386	a	Q413	b	Q440	a
Q360	a	Q387	a	Q414	c	Q441	a
Q361	d	Q388	a	Q415	c	Q442	a
Q362	a	Q389	b	Q416	a	Q443	a
Q363	a	Q390	a	Q417	d	Q444	a
Q364	d	Q391	a	Q418	a	Q445	b
Q365	b	Q392	a	Q419	d	Q446	c
Q366	d	Q393	a	Q420	a	Q447	c
Q367	d	Q394	d	Q421	d	Q448	c
Q368	d	Q395	b	Q422	a	Q449	c
Q369	d	Q396	a	Q423	a	Q450	b
Q370	a	Q397	d	Q424	a		
Q371	d	Q398	d	Q425	a		
Q372	a	Q399	b	Q426	b		
Q373	d	Q400	a	Q427	a		
Q374	a	Q401	b	Q428	a		
Q375	a	Q402	d	Q429	d		
Q376	a	Q403	c	Q430	b		
Q377	c	Q404	a	Q431	a		
Q378	b	Q405	a	Q432	a		

BIBLIOGRAPHY & REFERENCES

*J*nana Yoga, Bhakti Yoga, Karma Yoga, Raja Yoga- Swami Vivekananda

Hatha Yoga Pradipika - Swami Muktibodhananda Gheranda Samhita

Shreemad bhagwat Gita

Anatomy and Physiology of Yogic Practices Yogic Sukshma Vyayama

Asana, Pranayama, Mudra & Bandha Surya Namaskara

Kalyana

Patanjali Yoga Sutra

Yoga and Modern Psychology Management of Diseases

Yoga Teacher Manual for School teacher Teaching method for Yogic practices

www.ingramcontent.com/pod-product-compliance
Lightning Source LLC
LaVergne TN
LVHW091655070526
838199LV00050B/2177